RETURN to an Order of the Honourable the
House of Commons dated 13th May, 1974 for

D1743764

Report of the Committee of Inquiry into South Ockendon Hospital

Ordered by The House of Commons *to be printed*
14th May, 1974

LONDON
HER MAJESTY'S STATIONERY OFFICE
£1.30 net

ISBN 0 10 212475 2

FOREWORD BY THE SECRETARY OF STATE FOR SOCIAL SERVICES

In publishing this report I would like to thank Mr. Inskip and his Committee for the care they have devoted to their task and for the clear light they have shown on some disturbing incidents and on certain features of the administration of South Ockendon Hospital. I shall discuss the report and the action it recommends with the Regional and Area Health Authorities and I am proposing to refer its findings also to the General Nursing Council for their consideration.

Certain complaints by a nurse about nursing standards in Willow Villa between December 1971 and February 1972 led most directly to my predecessor's decision to set up the Inquiry. The Committee's conclusion is that during this period care of patients seldom exceeded in this villa the bare minimum and often fell below it, and that out of ten specific complaints concerning this villa six were fully and three partly justified. The decision to appoint this Inquiry was also influenced by the suspicions expressed in Parliament about the circumstances of the death of the patient Robert Robertson early in 1969. The Committee have shown that there was a number of unsatisfactory features about the available evidence, but they were not able to reach any sure conclusion on how he received the injuries from which he died. They were satisfied however that no other enquiries or proceedings would enable a sure conclusion to be arrived at.

The Report suggests that—although " the enormous majority of the staff at South Ockendon have worked very hard to care for their patients "—there were serious shortcomings in some wards in the standard of care, the Hospital Management Committee's management was weak, their methods of handling complaints and investigating untoward occurrences very unsatisfactory and their view of their own responsibilities too narrow. I accept these conclusions.

In reading this Report however it is important to have two things in mind. First the Committee identify as open to criticism what they see as a general unwillingness to intervene in practices in the Hospital which were held to be matters of individual clinical responsibility. This is an aspect in which there have been major changes in attitude, and changes in the understanding particularly of the role of doctors in the field of mental handicap, since the period in which most of the incidents investigated took place. Secondly I believe that criticism should be directed less at individuals who have had to work at South Ockendon under very difficult conditions, or at those who have had to try to deal directly with the problems arising from these conditions, than at successive Governments who have failed to ensure that NHS authorities devoted adequate resources to hospitals for the mentally handicapped.

Both the previous Government and its predecessor have sought to improve these services, and it was the late Mr. Richard Crossman whose new drive, launched in 1968, laid much of the groundwork for the Command Paper " Better services for the Mentally Handicapped" published in June 1971. These efforts have produced significant improvements. For example, capital expenditure of Regional Hospital Boards on hospitals for the mentally handicapped has increased by more than 60% in real terms since 1968/69 and expenditure per in-patient week, also in real terms, by more than a third. Nationally nurse staffing has increased by about a third and overcrowding had been reduced by a third between the beginning of 1970 and the end of 1971 and should by now be more than halved. Many visitors to hospitals for the mentally handicapped have also commented on the marked changes in atmosphere and environment as compared with a few years ago.

South Ockendon, as the Committee recognised, has shared in these improvements and it is right therefore to acknowledge the part played by its management and staff in the improvement which continues to take place there. Nevertheless I am by no means satisfied that standards are everywhere as high as I would want to see them. I am accordingly asking the new Health Authorities to review once again the standards of care and management in all their long stay hospitals, to ensure that a fair share of resources is allocated to them and to provide further opportunities for their staff to familiarise themselves with best practice. I shall also warmly commend to these authorities the Committee's observation that "all people charged with the management of a hospital, whether layman or professional, must have faith in their judgment and in the evidence of their own eyes. If they feel that something is wrong they must ask questions until they are satisfied. If they are not satisfied they must take appropriate action".

I will comment on only two other issues raised in the Report—

a. The Committee note that in Beech Villa the problems of overcrowding and understaffing had been compounded by concentration of difficult patients. This was not a situation unique to South Ockendon and indeed formed an important part of the difficulties studied by the Farleigh Hospital Committee of Inquiry which reported in 1971 following incidents at that hospital roughly contemporaneous with the incidents in Beech Villa which the Committee investigated in detail. Following the Inquiry at Farleigh Hospital preliminary advice was issued on the care of violent and difficult patients and Boards were asked in allocating resources to pay particular attention to situations which are potential sources of violence. Since then the National Association for Mental Health consultative document " Guidelines for the care of patients who exhibit violent behaviour in mental and mental sub-normality hospitals " has been published and my Department is now preparing jointly with the Royal College of Psychiatrists and the Royal College of Nursing formal advice for authorities, doctors and nurses.

b. The Committee draw attention to the attitude to criticism shown by management and senior staff at the hospital. Too often there was a closing of ranks instead of the objective inquiry properly called for. I have no doubt that a factor in this was a highly laudable feeling of the need to keep the team together in tackling difficulties to which the hospital's resources were recognised to be inadequate. But the result, inevitably, was dulling of sensitivity to matters which had clearly gone wrong. It is unlikely that some of the difficulties, for example in Cypress Villa when it served as a Security Unit, would have developed so far as they did had the Hospital Management Committee's own arrangements for investigating complaints been more satisfactory. In this connection I understand that the Davies Committee on Hospital Complaints Procedure took account of relevant evidence taken by the South Ockendon Inquiry at their public hearing.

BARBARA CASTLE,
Secretary of State for Social Services.

The Rt. Hon. Sir Keith Joseph, Bt. M.P.,
   Secretary of State for Social Services

Dear Sir Keith,

   We have held the inquiry into the care of patients at South Ockendon Hospital, South Ockendon, Grays, Essex, and I now submit our report which we have all signed.

                    Yours sincerely,

                                  signed J. HAMPDEN INSKIP
                                          Chairman

MEMBERS OF THE COMMITTEE OF INQUIRY

Mr. J. Hampden Inskip, Q.C.   Recorder of the Crown Courts, Chairman.

Mr. H. McCree, S.R.N., R.N.M.S.   Chief Nursing Officer, Coldeast and Tatchbury Mount Group Hospital Management Committee, Southampton.

Mrs. Patience Sheard, C.B.E., J.P., B.A.   Alderman, Sheffield County Borough Council.

Dr. E. W. Shepherd, M.B., B.S., D.P.M., M.R.C.S., L.R.C.P., F.R.C.Psych.   Physician Superintendent, Leavesden Hospital, Abbots Langley, Watford.

Sir John Wills, Bt., T.D., F.R.I.C.S., J.P., D.L.   Alderman, Somerset County Council.

Secretary Mrs. E. G. Croft

Assistant Secretary Miss C. M. Baines

CONTENTS

Appendices

CHAPTER I

INTRODUCTION

1. In February 1972 reports appeared in some newspapers that the police were investigating the death of an elderly patient in Willows Ward at South Ockendon Hospital. A few days later a State Enrolled Nurse, Mrs. Youell, who had worked on the night shift in Willows Ward tendered her resignation to the Hospital Management Committee and made serious allegations of unprofessional conduct and low nursing standards against one of the charge nurses of that ward. At the same time there was continued uneasiness in some quarters about earlier incidents at the hospital. In early March 1972 *The Sunday Times* and *The Guardian* published articles in which they reported that AEGIS (Aid for the Elderly in Government Institutions) was calling for a Government inquiry into the circumstances of the death of a young patient, Robert Robertson, in Beech Ward in February 1969. A fellow patient had been charged with his manslaughter and found Not Guilty, after the Prosecution had offered no evidence against him. It was alleged, therefore, that the mystery of the circumstances in which Robert Robertson received the injuries from which he died remained unsolved. There had been a still earlier incident, in 1968, when a young patient was found with injuries suggesting a severe beating. All these matters were raised in the House of Commons on 11 April 1972, when the Secretary of State was asked whether he would institute a Government inquiry. Mention was also made of an autistic boy who was said to be deteriorating rapidly in a locked side room at the hospital.

2. At this time the Hospital Management Committee had already set up an inquiry into Mrs. Youell's allegations but they soon concluded that an independent inquiry would be more appropriate and on 27 April the Secretary of State announced his decision to set up an independent and wider inquiry under Section 70 of the National Health Service Act 1946. The Terms of Reference were to enquire into the care of patients at South Ockendon Hospital and make recommendations.

3. The members of the Committee of Inquiry were appointed during May and we started work at once. Letters were sent to the nearest relatives of all who had been patients in South Ockendon Hospital at any time since 1 January 1968, asking them to get in touch with our Secretary if they felt they had any information or held any views that would assist us in our task. Similar letters were sent to all those who had been members of the Hospital Management Committee or on the staff of the hospital at any time since 1 January 1968. Other letters inviting information, or help in putting us in touch with others who could give information, were sent to the League of Hospital Friends and other voluntary organisations connected with the hospital, to AEGIS and to certain MPs who had shown particular interest in the care of patients at the hospital. In all some 3,200 letters were sent and we received 253 replies.

4. Under our directions members of the Treasury Solicitor's Department assembled the relevant documents, interviewed witnesses and took statements

from them. We had the assistance of Counsel, Mr. J. A. C. Spokes and Mr. M. J. L. Brodrick.

5. We met in public for the first time on Friday, 30 June 1972 in order to indicate the path we intended to follow and to give directions. Our Chairman then said:

"The terms of reference which I have read are very wide and we wish to indicate at this stage the provisional course that the Committee intends to follow. It is our present intention to concentrate on the period from 1 January 1968, but it will be necessary to look at earlier years in so far as problems may have been inherited from them, or created by the action or inaction during that time. It may be necessary to consider incidents that may have occurred before 1968. We will, of course, hear evidence about all incidents where it is alleged that the care of any patient has fallen below an acceptable standard. But also, and just as important, we intend to inquire into the care of the patients generally in all its aspects. It may be suggested that the care of the patients in this hospital, as in many similar hospitals, is made even more difficult than it would otherwise be by overcrowding and understaffing, and we intend to commence our inquiry at ward level because it is probably here more than anywhere else that such pressures are most felt. We wish to hear evidence from members of the staff and voluntary workers who work in the wards. How do they understand their job? What do they find to be good? How can they be helped to improve the quality of their care? In what ways, if any, do they feel unsupported? How can staffing shortages be overcome? We wish to hear evidence from the relations of patients who are or have been in the hospital, and indeed from former patients themselves. From this starting point we will work upwards. If the care given to patients is less than we feel it should have been, we will want to find out what has gone wrong; we will want to hear what problems the Regional Hospital Board and Hospital Management Committee have had in overcoming difficulties involved in the care of patients, in its widest meaning, and the steps they have taken or endeavoured to take to overcome them. In so far as the care of patients depends on, or will depend on, co-operation between the Regional Hospital Board, the Hospital Management Committee and the Social Service Departments in the hospital catchment area for the control of admissions and to provide alternative accommodation for patients who do not require hospital care, we will want to hear what has been done, what difficulties have been experienced, and what steps can be taken or can reasonably be taken to overcome them".

6. All evidence was heard in public. After the preliminary hearing on 30 June, we met in public to take evidence on 29 other days between 1 August and 13 November. Oral evidence was given by 116 witnesses; the transcript of evidence amounted to about 1,083,000 words.

7. Our Chairman in his opening statement announced that leave to be represented before us by Counsel or a solicitor would normally be granted to any person who appeared to us to be in some peril of censure or an adverse finding in regard to matters which we were investigating. Nine Counsel or solicitors represented authorities and individuals in the Inquiry. Mr. Spanswick, Assistant General Secretary of the Confederation of Health Service Employees, represented other staff in the hospital who were members of his Confederation.

8. We spent five days at South Ockendon Hospital. On two of these we heard evidence. On the other three days we visited various parts of the hospital. Two of our members visited a ward early in the morning and spoke to the night staff. During our visits we followed no pre-arranged course and were unaccompanied by any member of the staff. We talked freely to the staff about their work, but our report takes account only of what we saw at the hospital and of the evidence given on oath or in writing, together with the various hospital records, minutes of meetings etc. which were made available to us. Members of the Hospital Management Committee joined us for lunch at the hospital on 31 July, but this was entirely a social occasion and the subject matter of the Inquiry was not discussed. On 28 September we had lunch with the patients and staff in Poplars Villa and tea with those of Gloucester Drive.

9. In our report patients are referred to by initials, except where relatives have indicated their willingness for the patient's name to be used or where previous publicity has revealed his identity.

10. It will be convenient at this point to outline the background to some of our conclusions in order that we explain the course and content of our report.

11. Overcrowding, understaffing and lack of money have been the ground base to all work in the hospital for at least ten years. In the 1960s the hospital was urged to increase the number of patients in the hospital above that recommended by the Ministry of Health's space standards in order that hospital places could be given to those who urgently needed them. The effects of the overcrowding and understaffing became worse as the proportion of heavily dependent patients increased. The real weight of the burden was carried, as it always will be, by the staff working in the villas.

12. Declarations of policy and recommendations to improve the subnormality services have gone out from the Department of Health during these years. They are admirable documents with admirable aims and well thought out recommendations as to how they should be put into practice. But the gulf between the admirable goal and the money provided has seemed to the staff, and others, to be very wide. It has been fundamental to these plans that local authorities should provide hostels which would help to reduce overcrowding in hospitals as well as meet the needs of those still living with their own families, and there has grown up amongst many who work at South Ockendon Hospital an unhelpful but inevitable cynicism as they have observed that the exhortation has been unaccompanied by sufficient money to do more than scratch the surface of the need. In some ways it may even have led to a state of mind that plans for a bright future are more important than present action.

13. The enormous majority of the staff at the hospital have worked very hard to care for their patients. Many have come in to help patients and organisations in their off duty hours because they care very deeply about the patients and their work. Many have helped in making the villas more homely by providing various items to brighten the rooms. Others have worked with the Hospital Friends to raise money for equipment that is essential but which without their efforts could not have been bought. But they have struggled to achieve their best in grossly unfair circumstances. The staff/patient ratio meant that in many villas they could only give basic physical care. The occupational equipment was inadequate, leadership and guidance were often lacking. This has contributed to the sur-

prising variations in the standards of care in the hospital. With some exceptions the standard has been lowest in villas which have posed the greatest problems for their staff.

14. When day after day, month after month and year after year, there are too few staff working in inadequate accommodation, with inadequate facilities to look after too many severely subnormal and frequently overactive and incontinent patients, there will come a time when some will lose their self control and react to patients with varying degrees of violence. There will be others whose thresholds are imperceptibly lowered so that their standard of care declines. So we have found at South Ockendon Hospital.

15. The history of one of the villas, which was intended for medium security, revealed a decline to a wholly unacceptable and completely unjustifiable way of life. The intentions of the consultant were good; he made no secret of what he was doing; but he lacked the experience to carry out the very difficult job required of him. He needed clear guidance from the Regional Hospital Board, but did not receive it; he required close questioning about his actions and intentions when the early fruits of the unjustifiable regime began to appear, but he seems to have proceeded on his way without challenge. We have seen in the history of this villa all the stultifying effects that can flow from an unimaginative subservience to the doctrine of the clinical autonomy of the consultant. The patients undoubtedly suffered because of it.

16. Statistically the level of overcrowding and understaffing had been the same for several years. The Hospital Management Committee had been protesting to the Regional Hospital Board about the overcrowding throughout the 1960s; but it was only after the death of Robert Robertson following severe internal bruising in 1969 that the risk to patients and the grossly unfair stresses on staff from such conditions were recognised. Why were the warning signals not recognised and acted upon earlier? We try to answer this question.

17. When we have to report on allegations of violence and bad nursing we deal with the evidence and the reasons for our findings in some detail as it seems to us important that people, particularly those concerned, should know and be able to understand what we have found and why.

18. When dealing with the medium security villa we have again set out much of the evidence about the clinical autonomy of the consultant, using where possible the words of the witnesses. It seems to us essential to understand the attitudes in order to recognise the problems they create.

19. Where possible we have set out the events and our conclusions about them in chronological order. For some readers this will be a disadvantage, for it means that they will not be able to find all the matters relevant to one aspect of care in one section. We believe, however, that the chronological pattern of the report will permit the less impatient reader to follow through and ponder with us the events as they occurred and understand more clearly the basis for the suggestions we make in Chapter X which we have called "The Creation of a Home".

20. In all our work, from beginning to end, we have received great assistance from our Secretary, Mrs. E. G. Croft and from our Assistant Secretary, Miss C. Baines. Each has guided and encouraged us in her own way.

CHAPTER II

SOUTH OCKENDON HOSPITAL

History

21. South Ockendon Hospital was built by West Ham County Borough Council in the early 1930s. The village of South Ockendon, then well in the country, is now very near to the industrial sprawl along the Essex bank of the Thames, but it is still predominantly rural. The hospital itself with gardens and playing spaces cover 84 acres, but a further 98 acres of hospital land is farmed. It is remote from the London Boroughs from which the majority of its patients come.

22. The wards of the hospital are in villas, some of two storeys, some single-storied. In most cases one villa houses one ward, but one two-storey villa has been divided into two wards, one on each floor. The villas are separated by areas of grass, trees and paths. On a sunny day the appearance of the hospital is quite attractive with many of the patients sitting or playing out of doors. Even in winter the separated villas have a pleasantly uninstitutional aspect and some of them also create a homely atmosphere inside.

23. The original scheme provided for 750 beds and, at the outbreak of war in September 1939, nine wards, providing 520 beds, had been completed, together with buildings for recreation, workshops, staff residences, administration offices and central kitchen and laundry.

24. Since the start of the National Health Service in 1948, eleven new villas have been built, including the Gloucester Clinic (a treatment centre containing operating theatre, dental suite, physiotherapy, pathology laboratory, pharmacy, X-ray department and ancillary rooms as well as beds for 38 patients) and Cypress Villa (designed as a security unit but now providing accommodation for disturbed men patients). Several of the older villas have had major or minor upgrading and one prefabricated ward has been added to an existing villa. The number of available staffed beds reached a peak of 1065 in 1968 but by December 1971 had been reduced to 955. There have been a number of new buildings and extensions to provide or extend accommodation for occupational therapy and industrial therapy, a patients' school, staff residences, a nurse training school, recreational facilities, a psychology department and various central services. Certain services, particularly catering, laundry, heating, training and recreation, have not expanded to the same extent as the number of patients.

25. South Ockendon Hospital is the largest hospital in the South Ockendon Group which consists of two large hospitals, (the other, of about 350 beds, at Leytonstone) and six small units, of which four fall geographically into the eastern part of the Group with South Ockendon Hospital as their centre. These four are Little Warley Lodge at Brentwood, New Lodge Hospital at Billericay, Duvals Hospital at Grays and Ramsey Lodge Hospital, a holiday home, at Harwich. The first three are under the nursing control of the Principal Nursing Officer of South Ockendon Hospital.

26. The Chairman of the South Ockendon Group Hospital Management Committee is Mr. W. A. Nichols. The Group offices are at Leytonstone House, well to the eastern side of the Group's area and nineteen miles from South Ockendon. The Group Secretary, Mr. Harrison, the Chief Nursing Officer, Mr. Andrews, and other Group officers have their offices at Leytonstone House. Dr. Dutton, Chairman of the Group Medical Executive Committee, who was, until January 1972, Physician Superintendent for the Group, has his office at South Ockendon Hospital and is thus separated from the Group officers. The Hospital Secretary Mr. Offord and the Principal Nursing Officer Mr. Heffernan, have their offices at South Ockendon.

27. All hospitals in the Group are for mentally handicapped patients. The only other group for mentally handicapped patients in the North-East Metropolitan Region is the Royal Eastern Counties Group. Little Highwood, a small hospital for the mentally handicapped which first admitted patients in January 1971, is administered by the Brentwood Hospital Management Committee, a predominantly general group.

Statistics

28. Statistics of staff and beds at South Ockendon Hospital and the ratio between them, and similar statistics for all hospitals for the mentally handicapped in England and Wales are given in Appendix 3. They show that this hospital has for some years had more than the average number of medical and nursing staff: the number of qualified nursing staff in relation to patients is also above the national average. We do not derive any great assistance from these statistics for the national average is certainly not an acceptable level of staffing. We do not know the extent to which the other hospitals for the mentally handicapped are understaffed or the standard of care they provide.

29. Several of those who gave evidence to us had the impression that South Ockendon Hospital had a higher than average proportion of patients with aggressive behaviour disorder and severe physical handicap, though they were unable to provide evidence in support of this opinion. Subsequently, at our request, the Department of Health and Social Security supplied us with information taken from the Census of Mentally Handicapped Patients in Hospital in England and Wales at the end of 1970. This confirmed that the hospital did indeed have a higher than average proportion of heavily handicapped patients. $77 \cdot 3\%$ of all the patients in the hospital fell into the category of severe mental handicap as compared with an average in hospitals for the mentally handicapped in England and Wales of $71 \cdot 8\%$. Appendix 4 shows that the proportion of non-ambulant patients, of severely incontinent patients and of patients requiring much help to feed, wash and dress was, in each case, substantially above average, though to a smaller extent. But because of recruiting difficulties the staff was in all the years from 1968 until 1972 well below the establishment recommended by the Regional Nursing Officer.

The Development of Overcrowding

30. In 1948 Local Authorities were relieved of their responsibility for the provision of mental deficiency hospitals. This was taken over by the Minister of Health.

31. In 1959, following the Report of the Royal Commission on the Law Relating to Mental Illness and Mental Deficiency 1954–7 (Cmnd. 169) the responsibility for providing residential care for people not requiring hospital treatment was returned to the local authorities, but a substantial part of the cost of these hostels has had to come from rates and the progress in their provision has been extremely slow. This has meant that the hospitals have had to continue to accept patients on social grounds whether or not they strictly require hospital treatment. During the 1960s the numbers of severely handicapped children who survived into adult age increased and many more severely handicapped people lived on into old age. These trends greatly increased the numbers of heavily dependent patients in hospitals.

32. In 1960 the group catchment area was increased and the population it served increased from 879,000 to 1,465,500. In the same year the Board produced its ten year plan for inclusion in "A Hospital Plan for England and Wales" (Cmnd. 1604) which was published in January 1962. If it had been carried out, the problem of overcrowding would have been solved very much more quickly. Unfortunately the massive programme was undercosted by the Board and sharply rising building costs ate further into the money available for its implementation. As a result only a small part could be carried out. In deciding what cuts to make in its programme the Board took too optimistic a view of the number of hostels for mentally handicapped people that would be provided by the local authorities.

33. The only alternative was to increase the number of patients in hospitals. This policy was pursued at South Ockendon in spite of protests from the Hospital Management Committee, the Physician Superintendent and the nursing staff. By 1968 the level of overcrowding, judged against the Ministry's standard of 60 square feet of bed space for each person, was about 30%. Between 1964 and 1969 the money spent by the Board on the maintenance of its buildings was well below the national average as sums earmarked for this purpose had to be diverted to more pressing needs. This was one of the sources from which money might have been provided for the upgrading of out of date villas.

34. Throughout the 1960s the numbers of staff were very low. In 1965, for example, there were 262 nursing staff and 76 domestic staff to look after nearly 90 more patients than were cared for by 372 nursing staff and 64 domestic staff in 1972 (the staff figures given are whole time equivalents).

35. Although the level of overcrowding remained static from about 1963 to 1968, the increasing dependency of the patients added to the burden on the staff who were already too few in number.

HR—B

CHAPTER III

THREE CHILDREN

36. All the incidents referred to at the beginning of Chapter I and several others which came to our notice occurred in three villas, Beech, Cypress and Willows. We deal with the events in these villas in Chapters IV, V and VI, but first we propose to relate the effect of conditions in the hospital on the lives of three patients, who were admitted as children. Although they entered the hospital several years before 1968 their experience, which unfortunately is not unique, forms a useful bridge leading us into the five year period on which we have concentrated. We are able to see in their stories how a shortage of money leading to inadequate facilities and overcrowding led to a decline in their condition, anxiety for their parents and frustration for the staff who sought to care for them.

Patient V

37. Patient V was born on 23 January 1949. He suffered cerebral trauma at birth and developed epilepsy at an early age. He is spastic and severely subnormal. He was placed in a Spastic Unit in 1954 but owing to his mental incapacity he was unable to benefit from the teaching. In 1957 he joined a Training Centre where there was some initial improvement in his behaviour and concentration. Unfortunately the epileptic attacks increased and during the disturbed period following each attack he was aggressive and spiteful to other children. His parents had no alternative but to withdraw him from the Unit. In 1960, an attempt was made to get him into an establishment run by the National Spastics Society but this failed because of his low IQ of 35. That Society in a report dated 25 July 1960 stated that Patient V:—

   i. had epileptic episodes daily;

   ii. was ambulant with a fairly normal gait and considerable control of his hands;

   iii. had some speech that was clear;

   iv. had the behaviour pattern of a grossly retarded boy and would eventually need to be placed in a suitable hospital for severely subnormal children.

38. In 1959 Patient V spent a short time in South Ockendon Hospital but his parents removed him complaining of the conditions. By June of 1961, however, both parents recognised that their son needed hospital care and he was again admitted to South Ockendon Hospital where he remained until April 1971, when he was transferred to Little Highwood.

39. During the greater part of the ten years that Patient V was in South Ockendon Hospital his parents by letters to the hospital, the Press, their Member of Parliament and the Secretary of State conducted a campaign against the conditions in which their son had to live as a result of overcrowding and understaffing. We consider their complaints in detail at a later stage, but we emphasise at this stage that although their campaign was conducted with vigour their criticism was not aimed at the staff, who they accepted did their very best, but

against the unfair conditions in which they had to work. We accept that these parents were always sincere and motivated solely by a burning desire to improve the circumstances in which their son had to live. The language of their campaign became more biting as they became increasingly frustrated at their inability to bring about the improvements that everyone knew were desirable.

40. At the time of his admission Patient V was under Dr. Dutton who was then a consultant. Unfortunately the assessment form which should then have been completed was left with many blanks so that it is not possible to tell whether any proper assessment was made or what it revealed. It seems to have been the exception rather than the rule at this period for the assessment forms to have been completed on admission. It is therefore impossible from the hospital records to find any clear account of the patient's ability and condition at that time. Dr. Dutton thought that the report of the Spastics Society in July 1960 represented the patient's condition on admission to South Ockendon. He is now doubly incontinent, but we do not know if he was then. His father had reported to the Spastics Society that his son could feed himself if his food was cut up and could drink from a cup and that he was toilet trained in the morning and evening.

41. There is no doubt that Patient V deteriorated while he was at South Ockendon Hospital. He was admitted to Hawthorns Villa because it was considered that a single-storey building would be an advantage in view of his difficulty in walking. But this was soon realised to be unsuitable because in Dr. Dutton's words " he obviously required more stimulation, being the only person in that ward who could move about very much and talk". He was moved to Limes Villa which was also unsuitable because it was a two-storey building which contained a number of boisterous boys who were apt to knock into him. Thereafter he was in Briars Villa and, at times, the Gloucester Clinic.

42. In a report dated 11 March 1969 Dr. Dutton stated that Patient V was unable to stand or walk without support and that he had no useful speech and could not even indicate his wants in gestures. Dr. Dutton said in evidence that he thought that the decline in mobility was due to the fact that he was kept in a chair for long periods because of the danger of him falling over and injuring himself, particularly during fits. We find that this was the probable explanation for this deterioration. There were too many patients and too few staff in each ward for the patients to receive more than minimal care. The risk of injury from falling in a fit, or being pushed over, could only be removed by enforced inactivity which carried with it the risk of loss of mobility. Moreover patients who sat about reduced the chaos. We find that Patient V's speech deteriorated through lack of opportunity and of encouragement to use it.

43. Since Patient V was transferred to Little Highwood he has been encouraged to walk and has regained some mobility. His posture has improved when sitting, and his attention can be held for longer periods. But so far there is no improvement in his speech. His parents are pleased at the change and find him happier. This, however, has been achieved because he is in a much smaller unit of twelve patients with a higher staff ratio. The cost per week is much higher.

44. While he was at South Ockendon Hospital Patient V sustained the following injuries:—

21 July 1961   A graze of the left eyebrow caused by falling in a fit.

9

27 August 1961	Bruising of the right side of the chest caused by falling against a table in a fit.
15 September 1962	Bruising and slight skin loss over sacrum caused by falling in a fit.
15 October 1962	Inflammation of the tip of the left little finger, possibly as a result of being caught in a door.
12 January 1963	A burn from the left scapula to the left iliac crest probably as a result of leaning against a hot radiator.
7 March 1964	A cut beside the left eyebrow caused by falling in a fit.
4 June 1964	Deep lacerations requiring six stitches in the lobe of the left ear caused by a bite by another patient.
17 July 1964	Abrasions to right leg and arm and a broken foot caused by falling.
5 August 1964	Lacerations on the head. These were caused when another patient hit him and required three stitches.
27 August 1964	A slight graze over the left eye caused in a fall.
1 March 1965	Another patient tried to choke him but did no real damage.
21 June 1965	A cut on the back of the head caused by falling.
19 November 1965	A 'Y'-shaped laceration which required stitching on the head. Cause unknown.
3 May 1966	He was found lying in the yard with considerable bruising of the face and head. The injuries were consistent with him falling and then being trodden on.
17 October 1967	A cut on the head which required stitching caused by falling out of bed in a fit.
6 October 1968	A laceration over the right eyebrow caused when he was pushed over by another patient.
8 July 1969	Superficial bruising of spine. Cause unknown.

The Parents' Complaints

45.   i. The patient's notes reveal that on 19 November 1961 in the course of an interview the parents said that they were worried that their son was deteriorating and were told that this was likely to happen.

ii. In April 1963 the father complained that tall boys should not have to wear short trousers, that there was a shortage of socks, and that shortage of staff caused a delay of up to half an hour when parents came to see their children. Dr. Dutton in his letter of reply did not dispute the accuracy of the allegations.

iii. In January 1964 the father wrote complaining that on Sunday 19 January there were only 2 trainee male nurses and a ward maid on duty, and that his wife had to restrain one patient from hitting another. A report by the Chief Male Nurse showed that there were only 26 full-time staff and 5 part-time staff on duty that day to care for the hospital's 996 patients. Of these 31 only 9 were trained. Staffing shortages at that time were exacerbated by the Whitley Council's reduction in the working week and their ruling that qualified staff could not be paid overtime. This meant that qualified staff could only earn overtime by working their overtime hours in another hospital. Moreover there was a ban on recruiting nurses from a co-operative nursing agency. There are now many more staff at the hospital caring for fewer patients.

iv. On 23 November 1965 the father wrote to the Minister of Health complaining that he only discovered the injury of 19 November 1965 when he visited on the 21st. He further alleged that some patients had to stay in bed because there were not enough clothes. Dr. Matheson, the Physician Superintendent, wrote to Dr. Ramsay on 10 December 1965 accepting that on rare occasions the supply of clothes ran out, and it is noteworthy that Patient V's father stated that the position improved after his complaint. Dr. Matheson's letter, after summarising the position in regard to Patient V, continued " I cannot, however, emphasise too much that patients such as V should be cared for in much smaller units and with a much higher ratio of staff to patients. With due respect to Circular HM 65(104) the prospect of this kind of thing happening in even the foreseeable future seems remote. There was one frightening day a few weeks ago when on the male side there were only 2 staff per shift per villa and the average at the best of times is only approximately 3 per shift ".

v. In February 1969 patient V's mother wrote to the Management Committee and Local Press complaining that they had recently found a very bad scar running the whole length of their son's body, and that nobody in the hospital could explain how it happened. The father showed us a photograph of the scar, and we are satisfied that it is the scar from the burn which was caused on or about 12 January 1963. It is about 18 inches long and varies in width between 1 and 2 inches. Dr. Dutton thinks that it would have been a second degree burn requiring two-hourly dressings for weeks rather than days. There is no record of such dressings having taken place, neither is there any record of the parents having been notified of the burn. The parents certainly should have been notified, and we accept the father's evidence that this was not done. We do not understand why the parents failed to see the scar on any of their son's visits to his home in the intervening years, but this lapse of time explains why no explanation for the scar was immediately forthcoming when the parents started asking the staff about it in 1969.

vi. The father also stated that on one occasion when his son was in the Gloucester Clinic he found that a boil on his back had stuck to his jacket. We accept that this occurred, but emphasise that this is the only criticism of the Gloucester Clinic which has come to our notice. All the evidence indicates that it provides a consistently high standard of care.

Conclusions

46. i. Patient V needed a much smaller unit and higher staff ratio than South Ockendon could provide.

ii. The hard pressed staff did what they could for him while he was at South Ockendon, but it was not sufficient to avoid some deterioration

11

in his condition. This deterioration would probably not have occurred if he had been in a smaller unit.

iii. The parents refused to accept that nothing could be done to reduce the overcrowding and increase the staff. They made themselves unpopular with the management and staff of the hospital by drawing attention in strong language to some of the consequences of overcrowding and understaffing. They brought about some improvements.

iv. Patient V has improved since he moved to Little Highwood because he is in a much smaller unit with a higher staff ratio.

Patient VV

47. This patient was born on 27 June 1958 and was later admitted to Limes Villa in South Ockendon Hospital. In 1967 his parents complained to Dr. Dutton that he was bruised and excessively drugged and that they feared that he would deteriorate to the point of no return. Dr. Dutton informed them that the bruising was caused when their son fell out of bed, that a large ward was not suitable and that he wanted a special unit for the care of the psychotic child, but that this project had to be seen in the light of priorities and available funds. He did not deal with the allegation of excessive drugging.

48. The parents wrote to their Member of Parliament in December 1968 expressing great appreciation of the nurses but asking that a place be found for their son in an autistic unit and again suggesting that he was being given an excessive amount of drugs to the detriment of his health. On 13 December Dr. Dutton wrote to Dr. Ramsay saying " My sympathies I must admit are with Mr. VV. As you will remember on the occasion of the Regional Hospital Board's visit in 1966 I spelt out this problem in some detail, and I reiterated the need for facilities to cope with this sort of patient when they visited in September this year. VV is not the only child who is suffering in this way, and the pressures on staff with overcrowding and the extremely handicapped nature of the patients now being admitted means that physical care is often all that can be achieved. I am sorry that this is rather a depressing reply to your letter but nevertheless I cannot but be honest. We do have to use a fair amount of drugs in the control of these behaviour problems because it is impossible for the nurses who are pretty thin on the ground to give individual attention or to look after them in very small groups. . . . I feel that unless a considerable amount of money is spent increasing the physical standards for patients in hospitals for the mentally subnormal, this sort of condition and this sort of complaint from relatives will continue. You are as aware, I have no doubt, of the ideal situation in which to nurse these patients as I am, and I would personally like to see wards of considerably smaller size where we can endeavour to introduce a proper therapeutic atmosphere which is just not possible with the overcrowded conditions that now prevail ".

49. Dr. Dutton sent copies of this correspondence to Mr. Seaman who was then Chairman of the Hospital Management Committee. His covering letter commented " I am very sincere in my remarks about overcrowding and as you know this has concerned me for some time, and as I have stated in committee we are in fact doing positive harm to some patients. I feel that this letter is very pertinent. It is very remarkable in fact that the Regional Board have got away

with it for so long. I fully realise the difficulties that they face but with the greatly increased awareness of conditions in hospitals such as ours and the activities of the NAMH etc. I feel that we have not heard the last of this sort of challenge ".

50. At this time Limes villa contained 52 boys and male adolescents. There should have been 1 charge nurse and 5 other nurses on duty at all times during the day, but because of difficulties in obtaining staff and absence through sickness the average number of nursing staff on duty was 1 charge nurse and 2·31 other nurses. There should have been 3 domestics on the ward staff, but the average attendance was less than one.

51. Patient VV is still in Limes Villa which now has 40 patients. Dr. York-Moore, the consultant, informed us that VV's medication had been altered many times in an effort to find a drug regime which would help him and there was no question of over-medication. In the last year or so his condition, though fluctuating, had improved, largely as a result of concentrating staff resources on to a small group of difficult boys including VV.

52. These complaints by the parents of V and VV closely resemble the comments made by Dr. Dutton in a letter dated 6 December 1967 to Mr. Searle, the newly appointed Head of Nursing Services. He started by saying that he had for some time " been alarmed at the numbers of crimes committed in the name of staff shortage " and felt that it was time to try and " stop the rot before nurses really do become solely the custodians of the orifices ". He continued " You will remember in days gone by, nurses for the Mentally Subnormal were concerned with a lot of patient activities. Many of these have now been lost to the nurses, but even so, I feel that we have far too many patients on the wards doing nothing—we rely on tranquillisers rather than organised activities to control the patients. No longer are groups of severely subnormals taken out for walks to give them fresh air, and a healthy tiredness. The nursing staff do not involve themselves with kicking a ball about with the patients. Indoor activities are now non-existent. The 'square-eyed monster' takes the place of the leisure activities that staff and patients used to undertake. In my own mind, this has been a very retrograde step both for nursing and for patients. Could you, when you are considering the reorganisation of nursing, try to bring in some of these lost activities. I am sure the drug bill will go down, and both patients and staff will be healthier. Could we involve the Teaching Staff in such an idea—surely they could demonstrate to the students how to occupy the ' low grade ' patients —classes could play games with the patients and arrange various forms of exercise".

John Read

53. A picture of inactivity and deterioration was also described to us by Mrs. Read. Her son, John, a severely subnormal spastic, went to South Ockendon Hospital in 1955 when he was eleven years old. He spent about two years in Hawthorns, then about eight years in Limes and his last six years in Willows. He was transferred to Little Highwood in April 1971.

54. Mrs. Read was at all times satisfied with her son's " actual physical well-being ". Of the care given by the nursing staff she said " I think they gave their patients very good attention and I think that they did everything that they could

13

do in very, very difficult circumstances. It was hopelessly overcrowded ". Nevertheless, in spite of all that the staff could do, John's condition deteriorated. Mrs. Read thought that this occurred " because of overcrowding, mainly, because they just did not have the time to give to patients to stimulate them". Of the 57, or thereabouts, patients in Limes there were about 30 who were unable to feed themselves. On some Sundays when Mrs. Read visited her son she found two staff doing their best to cope.

55. When John was admitted to South Ockendon he had limited speech. After his admission staff told Mrs. Read that they never heard him say a single word. When she asked that he be given speech therapy and told the staff that he spoke when he came home she was informed that the numbers of staff were completely inadequate and they could not spend time on a child with such limited speech.

56. John was taken out for a walk every day before he went into South Ockendon and was then able to walk over a mile. He had worn leg irons until two years before his admission. Within a year of his entering South Ockendon his walking deteriorated, his knees turned inwards and his legs were no longer straight.

57. When Mrs. Read spoke to the staff about his inactivity " they said that they were so overcrowded that if a child would sit down they were only too thankful to leave him there ".

58. Mrs. Read joined the Friends of South Ockendon who made representations to the Hospital Management Committee about overcrowding. The attitude of the Management Committee and, indeed, the medical staff, to whom she spoke on two occasions, was that although they would see what could be done the situation would not improve until more accommodation was provided.

59. Mrs. Read said that when she visited John in Limes a few children were playing with educational toys. When he moved to Willows " there was a little more for them to do and one or two jigsaw puzzles and things like that. The standard of the patients seemed a little higher ".

60. Like Mr. V, Mrs. Read found that Little Highwood was a big improvement. She said his condition " has improved and he is now walking better, and he is also using educational toys and other things in that way. They say he is also using his initiative in getting up and walking about without being told to do so ". She attributes the improvement to the fact that there are only twelve patients in each villa with five staff to care for and help them. She added " There is definitely more space but also they are encouraged. The staff take them up to the town if they are going up to the town to buy some cigarettes. They just say ' Come on John ', or one of the others, and take them up there ". Unfortunately, however, John does not speak, and Mrs. Read has been told that it is not thought that speech therapy would be useful.

CHAPTER IV

BEECH VILLA

The Building and the Patients

61. Beech Villa is a two-storey pre-war building for high grade patients. At one time 76 such patients lived there. Upstairs there were, in 1968, three dormitories, two bathrooms, two WCs and one urinal and one side room. Downstairs there was one large day room with two smaller rooms at each end, six WCs and one urinal. (Four further siderooms, a downstairs bathroom and other sanitary accommodation were added in 1970). By the beginning of 1968 it was a closed (locked) villa for 61 severely subnormal patients. This was reduced to 52 by the Regional Hospital Board in May 1968 after pressure from Dr. Dutton. The normal number of staff on duty by day was one charge nurse, three other nurses and one ward orderly. Over 30 of the patients were incontinent. Any patient who defaecated downstairs had to be taken upstairs to the bathroom to be washed. If he struggled the nurses and the floor en route to the bathroom would often be scattered with faeces. 15 of the patients who were severely subnormal were kept by day in a locked room on the ground floor, known as the low grade room, with one member of the staff in constant attendance. There was very frequent violence involving attacks by patients on other patients and staff.

62. Dr. Harfst, the consultant responsible for the patients in Beech Villa, described how, on his arrival in September 1967, he discovered that it had been used as the dumping ground for aggressive and severely disturbed patients by the rest of the hospital. It was " overflowing with these patients " and the overflow was being distributed among the other wards. He said about half of the patients were known to be periodically disturbed and violent " and about a dozen of them were regularly violent, and the incidence of violence seemed to me to be really extreme, it occurred every day. Very often it was against members of the staff. Accident reports were coming in regularly. I do not think I have ever seen myself such concentrated violence in any situation. Certainly I have never seen anything like it in a special hospital, and it would never have been tolerated. I was surprised when I first came how this was accepted by the staff as being just part of their job and something which really could not be altered and there was no hope of altering it. They just went about their job. As time went by I gradually accepted it myself . . . ". Later he said that the whole hospital was affected by this acceptance and pervaded with the feeling that nothing could be done, although not to the same extent as in Beech Villa where the situation was more acute than anywhere else.

63. Mr. Large, a charge nurse in Beech Villa during 1968 and 1969, said " it was the most violent villa. It was like a dustbin for the rest of the hospital. What would happen was that if a patient on the ward became so violent that they could not control him . . . the answer would be ' Transfer to Beech '. After a few years you had patients nobody else could cope with, and instead of having just one you had fifty of them ". He added " The majority of these people are very active, very strong, they have no idea of their own strength ". In another part

of his evidence he gave this account of the violence: " they would get a man down and then they would do what they could. They would kick, they would stamp, they would hit each other over the head with chairs, they would try to strangle you. They strangled my opposite charge twice on the stairway. They threw him down a flight of stairs and he had a fractured femur. A Chinese staff nurse, Mr. Wong, had a suspected fracture of the jaw. Mr. Taylor was assaulted six or seven times, and his spectacles broken. I had a broken finger which is recorded ".

64. We have studied the patients' records and the injury reports and accept that these accounts of violence in Beech Villa are substantially accurate. In May 1969 the Post-Ely Working Party said of the patients in this villa, " They skirmished with each other, teased each other or tore at their clothes or remained withdrawn. The room was bare and cheerless with tables and chairs, but no material for activity at all. The 3 male nurses in the 2 rooms did their best to ' keep order ' ".

Patient GG

65. On the night of 16 to 17 June 1968 Beech Villa was left in charge of a student nurse, Mr. Powell, who was then 19 years old and in his first year of training, and a Nursing Assistant, Mr. Ramen, who had even less experience. One of the patients in the villa was GG, who was then 23 years of age. He is severely subnormal, suffers from epilepsy, is incapable of speech, doubly incontinent and defenceless.

66. We propose first to set out facts about which there was no dispute in the evidence before us:—

    i. When Mr. Large came on duty at about 7.00 a.m. on 17 June Mr. Powell reported to him that he had found some marks on GG. Mr. Large saw that there was no entry in the Night Report concerning GG and told Mr. Powell to make an entry in the Night Report to cover himself. Mr. Powell, who had previously made the entry " All patients appear well and comfortable at time of report ", then wrote " GG— Noticed to have wield [weal] marks on outer aspects of arm and thigh. Cause? ".

    ii. Mr. Large made out an Injury Report in the following terms:—
" Reported to myself at 7.00 a.m. on taking over ward that patient had various marks and bruises on his body, time of occurrence unknown, incident reported in night report ". He described the injuries as " 2 long weals on upper right arm, inflamed area on lower left trunk. One weal on (Rt.) buttock and 4 weals left leg. 8 weals on Rt. leg + 1 weal across lower abdomen near hairline ".

    iii. Mr. Large reported these injuries to the Assistant Chief Male Nurse, Mr. Wood, at about 9 a.m. He examined the patient and reported his condition to the Nursing Officer.

    iv. Mr. Large also reported patient GG's condition to Dr. Kant by telephone at about 10.00 a.m. He told him that more bruises had come out since he first saw the patient at 7.00 a.m.

16

v. Dr. Kant examined the patient at 11.30 a.m. and signed the injury report adding " many other lesions will be given in separate report ". The separate report which Dr. Kant then made out detailed the following injuries.

"A. Injuries of the Right Upper Arm
1. At the lateral side an extensive injury $7'' \times \frac{3}{4}''$.
2. A bruise with discolouration at the back.
3. Another injury of size $3'' \times \frac{3}{4}''$.

B. Right Forearm
A similar injury—one in front and one at the back a few inches above the wrist.

C. Right Lower Leg
8 transverse marks of similar type across the front and 4–5 transverse marks across the back.

D. Left Leg
2 transverse marks in front and 4–5 transverse marks on the back with a small bruise and discolouration.

E. A transverse mark on the left buttock $2'' \times \frac{1}{2}''$.

F. A transverse mark left upper arm at the back.

G. Few linear abrasions around the anal cleft.

H. A transverse mark on the lower abdomen just above the pubic hair line.

The Back
1. A punctate type of wound on the back just below the left scapula size $6'' \times 4''$.
2. Another punctate wound of smaller size on the lower part of the back ".

Dr. Kant extracted two bristles from the punctate wounds and left one in the wound in case further examination was required. He said in his report that all the injuries were probably inflicted by one object. " They all have the same shape and size. To describe one: there is an erythematous ring surrounding a clear patch of skin in the centre which obviously escaped the site of impact, suggesting a hole in the centre of the object used e.g. braces. All these lesions are running transversely suggesting that they are not caused by accident but probably inflicted not once but many times ". He went on to say that he thought the punctate wounds had been inflicted with a scrubbing brush.

vi. Dr. Kant had the patient removed to the Gloucester Clinic and sent his written report to Dr. Dutton who examined the patient at 2.00 p.m. and commenced enquiries.

vii. Dr. Dutton interviewed Mr. Powell at 4.30 p.m. that day. Mr. Powell told him that he had done his normal round of incontinent patients at 10.00 p.m., that he had got patient GG up and changed him and that, when he was stripped, he had noticed a mark on one of the patient's legs. He said that there was only a dim light and he had not noticed the other injuries until he got the patient up in the morning.

viii. Dr. Dutton then interviewed Mr. Ramen who told him that Mr. Powell had shown him the marks on the patient's right arm and back at 11.30 p.m. with the lights full on in the dormitory.

17

ix. In view of the conflict Dr. Dutton then saw both together, but each adhered to his version of events and made a short written statement which Dr. Dutton handed to the Police when he reported the incident to them at 5.30 p.m. that day.

x. Police Constable Lynch interviewed Mr. Powell at the hospital at 7.15 p.m. on 17 June. Student Nurse Powell initially said that the statement he had made to the hospital authorities was the truth. When P.C. Lynch said that he wanted a fuller statement and cautioned him, he then said " No, wait, I want to change my story. The statement I made earlier is a pack of lies ". He was asked why it was a pack of lies and said " Because I was covering for Ramen going to sleep last night and there was not a bed round done at 10.00 p.m., so I did not notice the marks until 6.00 a.m. this morning ". He then made a written statement in which he said that patient GG was asleep from the time he came on duty at 7.30 p.m., that he did no bed round at 10.00 p.m. and that he saw no marks on patient GG until he got him up in the morning at 6.00 a.m.

xi. Subsequent to making that statement Mr. Powell was questioned further, but we need only refer to part of the interview between him and Detective Sergeant Knight later that evening. The Detective Sergeant asked him why he had told the hospital authorities that he had found marks on patient GG's leg at 10.00 p.m. He replied " I was covering up for other people, I suppose ". It was then pointed out to him that he had not only on his own account shown the marks to Mr. Ramen in the morning, but had also reported them to Mr. Large. When he agreed that this was so the Detective Sergeant commented " Then in fact you were not covering up for anyone else because according to what you say, you brought it to the attention of at least two people ". Mr. Powell replied " The way it looks I am going to get into trouble for something I haven't done ".

xii. Police enquiries revealed the following facts which were not disputed before us:—

a. That the weal marks could have been caused by the handle of a bath brush that was kept at night in a locked bathroom to which only the staff had the key.

b. That the bristles from the punctate wounds were similar to the bristles in the bath brush.

67. We now turn to two pieces of evidence over which there was some area of disagreement.

68. In his report of 17 June 1968 Dr. Kant said " The patient, although he does not complain, is obviously in a lot of pain. He is extremely subnormal, epileptic, and is very frightened of my touching the wound or even reaching his back. His behaviour this morning seems to have changed suddenly into that of a very timid frightened man. He is usually a quiet chap sitting in his wheelchair without being a problem ". Dr. Dutton found the patient was exceedingly apprehensive of anyone behind him when he examined him at 2.00 p.m.

69. Mr. Wood, on the other hand, told us that at 9.00 a.m. the patient " appeared his normal self. He was not in any pain or stress ". Mr. Powell in his

evidence said that when he found the marks at 6.00 a.m. patient GG did not appear to be frightened or in pain. He said that if he had appeared to have been in pain he would have called someone.

70. We accept the evidence of Dr. Kant which is supported by his contemporaneous note. Mr. Wood had no such note to assist him and, although we are sure that he was trying to be accurate, we are satisfied that his recollection of events four years ago is at fault.

71. The second matter on which there was some dispute was over the time at which the injuries were caused. Mr. Powell said that the injuries might have been caused before he came on duty. In his report of 17 June 1968 Dr. Kant wrote at 11.30 a.m. " All these wounds have only a redness so far, not yet acquired the swelling, suggesting that these wounds are probably of less than 12 hours' duration ". In evidence before us he said that in his opinion the injuries were inflicted not earlier than 11.30 p.m. or later than 5.30 a.m. A Charge Nurse, Mr. Hardas, who was then a student nurse on the afternoon shift of 16 June, told us that he had changed patient GG's bedclothes and given him a night shirt at 7.30 p.m. and that he had seen no marks on his body then. It is not possible to be precise as to when the injuries were caused, but we are satisfied that it was well after 8.00 p.m.

72. Who caused the injuries to patient GG? We were unable to call Mr. Ramen to give evidence as he is overseas. We did, however, hear evidence from a patient, KK. Before deciding to call him to give evidence we had a report from Dr. Finn M.B., M.R.C.Psych., D.P.M., who said that this patient sees to all his own personal needs and that he can tell the time and read moderately well. His orientation in space and time is accurate and he can talk well on day to day affairs. He was able to name the Queen and the Royal Children and without prompting stated that Northern Ireland was a current area of strife. Patient KK regularly helps with the bathing of other patients in the villa. Mr. Wood in answer to the question by Mr. Powell's counsel, " He is not a very trustworthy person? " replied " Sometimes yes, sometimes no. It is difficult to tell ". Dr. Harfst, the consultant responsible for Beech Villa, regarded KK as capable of deliberately misreporting events around him to suit his own ends and would not regard him as a reliable witness of fact.

73. Patient KK told us that Student Nurse Powell and Nursing Assistant Ramen had found patient GG standing naked by his bed after wetting it and that they hit him with the bath brush and marked him. To begin with he said that Mr. Powell got the brush from the sluice and hit patient GG with it and then put it back in the sluice. While this was going on Mr. Ramen was helping Mr. Powell and trying to get patient GG back to bed. In cross-examination by Mr. Powell's counsel patient KK agreed that he had told the police that it was Mr. Ramen who did the hitting. He added " Mr. Powell hit him first and after that Mr. Ramen ".

74. Dr. Dutton in evidence said that he had interviewed patient KK on 17 June 1968 and that he had then said that Student Nurse Powell was in the office writing when GG was assaulted by a curly-headed nurse. Patient KK was in our opinion an unreliable witness.

75. Finally on this incident we heard the evidence of Mr. Powell. He said that his recollection was not clear after the lapse of four years but that the truth was

set out in his statement to the police. In cross-examination he was shown a statement he had made to Mr. Pratt from the Treasury Solicitor's Department in July 1972. He said he had refused to sign the statement because his memory was not good and he had told Mr. Pratt that the truth was in his statement to the police which he had not seen for four years. He agreed, however, that the statement accurately recorded what he had told Mr. Pratt: that on the night of 16 June he did a round of the patients between about 9.00 p.m. and 10.00 p.m., and that on this round it was the practice to change the night attire of incontinent patients who required changing, and that he was fairly sure that GG was out of bed at that time and naked. He added in his evidence " GG would do this if he was wet ". He agreed that he told Mr. Pratt he had noticed that patient GG had a large number of red marks on his body and that they were mainly on the upper part of his back and shoulder and some on his buttocks and that he could not remember whether there were any marks on the arms and legs. He further agreed that he had told Mr. Pratt " I think I showed the marks to Mr. Ramen, but I cannot now be sure. I cannot remember whether I washed GG or whether I put a nightshirt on him, but I remember that he went straight back to bed and went to sleep ".

76. Mr. Powell in cross-examination adhered to his evidence that the truth was contained in his statement to the police, namely that he saw no injury of any kind on patient GG until he got him up at 6.00 a.m. He agreed that what he had said to Mr. Pratt four years later was totally different, but sought to attribute this glaring discrepancy to a poor memory and difficulties in recollecting what he had tried to forget.

77. We have no hesitation in rejecting Mr. Powell's evidence. We are satisfied that none of his statements to the hospital authorities or to the police or to Mr. Pratt was truthful. It is important to consider the sequence of his statements together with his explanations for making them.

    i. At about 4.30 p.m. on 17 June 1968 he told Dr. Kant and the hospital authorities that he had noticed the mark on patient GG's leg at 10.00 p.m. when he was doing the bed round and that he had shown this to Mr. Ramen when he came up at about 11.00 p.m. He told us that he had made this untrue statement to cover up for Mr. Ramen going to sleep and for his own failure to do a bed round.

    ii. At about 7.15 on the same day he made a second statement in which he said that he had not seen patient GG out of bed at any time during the night and that he had seen no marks on him until he got him up at 6.00 a.m. He told us that he had made his second statement after he had realised that his first untrue statement to the hospital authorities had got him into trouble. When the police cautioned him he decided to tell the truth.

    iii. He said that when he gave his account to Mr. Pratt in July 1972 it was a lapse of memory which made him revert to the untrue statement and forget the contents of the truthful one.

78. If the second statement had contained the truth we are satisfied that Mr. Powell would have remembered, when interviewed by Mr. Pratt, that he had not seen any marks on patient GG until the morning. We are satisfied that the only explanation for the discrepancy between Mr. Powell's statement to the police

and his account to Mr. Pratt is that he was unable to remember which untrue story he had told to whom.

79. We are satisfied that Mr. Powell did not lie merely to save Mr. Ramen's alleged sleeping on duty or his own alleged failure to carry out a bed round from coming to the notice of the hospital authorities. We are satisfied that Mr. Powell took part in an assault on patient GG which caused the injuries found by Dr. Kant and that this assault was probably committed because he found patient GG had wetted his bed and was standing naked beside it. We were, as we have said, unable to hear evidence by Mr. Ramen and we are unable to say whether he took part in the assault.

80. Mr. Powell and Mr. Ramen were young and inexperienced. They should not have been left in charge of a difficult villa in which about 30 of the 51 patients were incontinent. The strain of trying to keep incontinent patients clean is great and self-control may be lost.

The Steps Taken by the Hospital

81. Following the discovery of the injuries to patient GG, Mr. Powell and Mr. Ramen were transferred to day duty under close supervision. The matter was reported to the Patients and Welfare Sub-Committee on 19 June, and on 21 June the two nurses were suspended from duty. On the same day a report was sent to the Ministry of Health and the Regional Hospital Board.

82. On 22 July the hospital was informed that the Director of Public Prosecutions had decided not to institute any proceedings. In the meantime the Hospital Management Committee had held disciplinary proceedings against Mr. Powell and Mr. Ramen on 2 July. They were each charged " That on the night of 16/17 June 1968 in Beech Villa you were grossly negligent in your nursing responsibilities concerning the care of GG ". The Chairman of the disciplinary committee was Mr. Nichols who is now Chairman of the Management Committee. Mr. Powell and Mr. Ramen were both found guilty of negligence, but so far as we can discover, neither the negligence alleged nor that found proved against them was ever particularised. It is not surprising that Mr. Powell got the impression, as he told us in evidence, that it was being alleged that he had struck GG, or that Mr. Ramen had struck him and he had not interfered. Even Mr. Nichols seems to have been misled as to the nature of the charges. He told us " I was privileged to chair this investigation, and here we had charges with regard to beating the boy with a brush on his buttocks ". We consider that whenever a charge of negligence is made against hospital staff the acts or omissions relied upon as constituting the negligence should be set out in the charge.

83. Mr. Powell was given and accepted the opportunity of resigning. Mr. Ramen was told that he would be redesignated as a ward orderly but he also resigned.

84. On 15 July 1968 the General Nursing Council received a notice of discontinuance of training for Mr. Powell. The reason given was that he was " entering HM Forces ". At the bottom of the document Mr. Hubbard, the Deputy Head of Nursing Services at South Ockendon Hospital, had signed on 11 July 1968 that the conduct of Mr. Powell had been " satisfactory on all counts ".

85. We cannot share Mr. Nichols' view of this incident expressed in his proof of evidence which was treated as his evidence in chief. " My impressions of this incident were that it was not a serious assault but contrary to good nursing practice. The Committee felt that the action taken was correct and that there were no lessons to be learned from this incident or further action to be taken, this being the first incident for several years ".

86. On 15 November 1968 Dr. Dutton outlined to the Group Medical Advisory Committee the problem of patient overcrowding and its attendant evils within the Group. The Committee agreed that its Honorary Secretary, Dr. Harfst, should write to the Hospital Management Committee " describing this very serious situation and expressing grave concern ".

87. Doctor Harfst wrote to Mr. Harrison on 13 January 1969. The delay of two months was unfortunate, but Dr. Harfst was an extremely busy man with a very heavy work load. The letter, which is to be found at Appendix 5, was clear and forceful. Nobody reading it could doubt that the Medical Advisory Committee felt that the position was very serious.

88. The Agenda for the next Hospital Management Committee meeting was sent out on 24 January 1969. It contained no reference to this letter or its contents. The Hospital Management Committee met on 31 January 1969 and Dr. Dutton, who was Chairman of the Medical Advisory Committee as well as Physician Superintendent, was in attendance. No mention was made of the letter, or its contents. The Agenda for the next meeting of the Hospital Management Committee was sent out on 21 February 1969 but once again no reference was made to this letter or its contents. Management Committee members appear to have been unaware of its existence until Dr. Dutton drew their attention to it during the meeting on 28 February 1969, and it was then resolved that it should be circulated to all members as soon as possible. By that time further unfortunate events had occurred in Beech Villa.

89. On 6 February 1969 Dr. Dutton wrote to Dr. Ramsay saying that he was staggered that they ran a service so cheaply when compared with long-stay or chronic sick patients. He continued "We do not spend as much on nursing care—medical care—training of nurses—feeding—heating and lighting—maintenance of buildings—general cleaning—and general portering as these other hospitals, and why anyone should assume that it is cheaper to keep a hospital for the subnormal (in fact the severely subnormal) clean as compared with a long-stay or chronic hospital is beyond my comprehension. Similarly, why it should be cheaper to feed our patients, or nurse them, or train nurses to look after them, is again quite incomprehensible, and as long as this sort of shoe string economy is applied to hospitals for the mentally subnormal, I am convinced we will continue to get trouble like the one we have recently been bothered with. It is of course worth pointing out that one of the ways costs are kept down is by this extensive overcrowding which is forced upon us and of course if we reduce the overcrowding the cost per inpatient week would rise markedly and probably bring us somewhere nearer to line with the costs of other types of hospitals. I realise this is none of your making but I feel that I must protest somewhere and other than sending them to someone like Mrs. Robb, I am not sure to whom I can protest ".

90. Dr. Dutton's fears were justified. On 20 February 1969 a patient, Robert Robertson, died of internal injuries sustained in Beech Villa. It was a pity that Dr. Dutton placed at the top of his letter of 6 February the words "*personal and in confidence*".

Patients HH, CC and DD

91. On the night of 19/20 February 1969 Mr. Knopp, a State Enrolled Nurse, and Mr. Crowson, a student nurse, were on duty in Beech Villa. Mr. Large was the Charge Nurse who took over from them in the morning. The circumstances in which Mr. Large came to work in the hospital are set out in paragraphs 355 to 357.

92. Mr. Crowson's evidence to us can be summarised thus:

i. The night staff normally commenced to get the patients up at about 6.00 a.m. With the exception of a very few patients who did domestic work, all the patients were normally kept upstairs until the day staff arrived. Sometimes, however, patients were taken downstairs by the night staff before the arrival of the day staff, but when this occurred all the patients were brought down as it was not usual to separate the staff as would be necessary if some patients were upstairs and some down. An important factor in whether the patients were taken downstairs before the day staff arrived was the time at which the day staff arrived on duty. If they arrived early the patients would probably all be upstairs.

ii. On the morning of 20 February Mr. Large arrived at the villa at 6.45 a.m. although his official time for taking over was not until 7.00 a.m. The patients were all upstairs with the exception of some of the ward workers. Mr. Crowson was standing in the neighbourhood of the door between the corridor outside the office and the adjoining dormitory keeping an eye on a group of the low grade patients who had congregated in that area. Mr. Large went into the office and then went round the dormitories with Mr. Knopp. Mr. Large returned shortly afterwards to find patient HH standing near the office door with a runny nose. He picked up a folded sheet from the linen trolly in the passage " and struck the patient, not very severely, across the face with it, wiping his nose ". He put the sheet back on to the trolley and went into the office. He did not know if Mr. Knopp saw this occur as he was not aware of him returning from the dormitories with Mr. Large. He might have delayed in a dormitory to speak to a patient or check a bathroom or lavatory.

iii. CC was another low grade patient who was waiting to be taken downstairs. He had the habit of chewing up draw sheets and on occasions had chewed through the brake cables of bicycles parked outside and through television wire. Two or three minutes after Mr. Large had struck HH with the sheet Mr. Large, Mr. Knopp and Mr. Crowson were talking in the office on the first floor when a patient called from the corridor that patient CC was chewing a draw sheet. Mr. Large went out into the corridor and found CC squatting in the corridor with his back to the wall chewing the draw sheet and tearing it into strips. Mr.

23

Large kicked CC in the face with the underpart of sole of his shoe and knocked CC's head against the wall. There was some redness on CC's cheek and a small trickle of blood coming from his mouth, consistent with him having bitten his tongue or injured the membrane inside his mouth. CC did not say anything as he is incapable of speech. Mr. Crowson was unable to say whether Mr. Knopp came to the office door and saw the incident.

iv. About two minutes after Mr. Large had kicked CC, he, Mr. Knopp and Mr. Crowson were in the office discussing a patient, DD, who was sitting or squatting on a chair in the office with his feet up on the chair. He was severely subnormal, incapable of speech and overactive, and had been admitted to Beech Villa from Limes Villa on the previous day. He had spent the night in the side room for assessment. While the three members of the staff were discussing the reason for his admission to Beech Villa, Mr. Large struck the patient across the bridge of his nose with a kind of chopping action with the side of his hand. When he was asked whether it was a hard blow Mr. Crowson said " it is difficult to judge. I think it was a reasonably hard blow. Certainly not with the full weight of the body behind it, but a reasonably hard blow. I think this is a particularly sensitive area and it would not need too hard a blow for it to be painful ... The patient cried out and his eyes watered ". Mr. Crowson said that Mr. Knopp must have seen this incident.

v. He went off duty at about 7.05 a.m. and returned to duty at about 12.55 p.m. the same day. Shortly after this he assisted Robert Robertson who had been found in a distressed condition in the dormitory. (We deal with the death of Robert Robertson in the next section of this report).

vi. In the course of the afternoon he told Mr. Shrimpton, a senior State Enrolled Nurse, about what he had seen that morning.

vii. The next evening following the death of Robert Robertson he, and other staff, were interviewed by the police. As he waited in the Administration block for his turn to be interviewed Mr. Knopp came out, and as he passed he said out of the side of his mouth " Nothing happened ". In his first statement made at 9.20 p.m. he said nothing about Mr. Large having assaulted HH, CC or DD, but he subsequently reconsidered things and made a second statement detailing these assaults at 10.00 p.m. the same evening.

93. Mr. Knopp's evidence did not agree with that of Mr. Crowson. He said that when Mr. Large came on duty at about 6.50 a.m. there were about 35 patients downstairs and that the rest were upstairs. Mr. Crowson was already downstairs with the low grade patients. He said that this was following his normal practice. He agreed, however, that two staff on duty in a villa should not be separated unless this was essential, that it was his duty to count the number of patients with Mr. Large before he went off duty and that he could not do this without leaving the patients upstairs unattended if some of the patients were downstairs and some upstairs. Later in his evidence he modified these replies by saying that he had only recently become aware of these rules or regulations. He denied that he had said to Mr. Crowson " Nothing happened ".

94. Mr. Maghoo, who is now a State Enrolled Nurse and was then a student nurse, arrived late on duty that morning between 7.05 and 7.10 a.m. It was his job to look after the low grade patients in the small room downstairs. He said that he went upstairs to get them and found that they were waiting for him in and near the corridor on the first floor.

95. Mr. Shrimpton's recollection was very confused, but he said that his statement made to the police at 4.20 p.m. on 22 February 1969 would have been correct. In that statement he said that at about 3.00 p.m. on 20 February Mr. Crowson had told him that Mr. Large had been in a temper when he came on duty that morning and that he had seen him hit CC across the nose. The statement continued " I don't think he mentioned anything about Mr. Large hitting any other patient ". In his evidence to us he said Mr. Crowson may have said that Mr. Large hit other patients. Mr. Shrimpton did not tell Mr. Crowson to report the matter and did not tell Mr. Davies, the Charge Nurse, what Mr. Crowson had said.

96. Dr. Jones, who was then a medical assistant at South Ockendon Hospital, said that in the course of his visit to Beech Villa between 12.00 noon and 1.00 p.m. that day he had been asked to examine DD who had been admitted from Limes Villa on the previous day. Mr. Large had told him that this patient's behaviour was very disturbed indeed, and that he was aggressive and very destructive to property and clothing.

97. Mr. Large denied that he had assaulted any patient, and said that when he arrived on duty most of the patients were downstairs with perhaps about twelve remaining upstairs.

98. On the afternoon of 22 February 1969 HH, CC and DD were examined by Dr. Dutton and no sign of injury was found on any of them.

99. It was urged on behalf of Mr. Large that the evidence of Mr. Crowson was not reliable because he suffers from epilepsy and because he himself has assaulted a patient. We gave careful consideration to these matters.

100. As to the epilepsy, we accept Mr. Crowson's evidence that he has had no fits since 1966, and that he controls it by anti-convulsant drugs. His epilepsy does not in our opinion affect his credibility as a witness. Evidently it was not thought by senior nursing staff to affect his competence as a nurse either, for he was made a staff nurse in June 1969 and a charge nurse in December 1970.

101. As to the assault by Mr. Crowson, at 8.15 a.m. on 15 January 1971, Mrs. Archer, an Assistant Matron, entered Poplars Villa and found Mr. Crowson verbally chastising a female patient after which he struck her face and kicked her buttocks. He said to Mrs. Archer " I can only say in mitigation of the circumstances that this is a particularly stressful time of day, but I do not offer this as an excuse ". On 18 January the patient was examined by Dr. Dutton but no marks from the assault could be found. Mr. Crowson was interviewed by Mr. Searle, the Head of Nursing Services, and by Mr. Andrews, the Chief Nursing Officer, and the matter was referred to the Hospital Management Committee who agreed that no action need be taken. Mr. Crowson remained as a charge nurse in Poplars Villa, and in 1972 the Hospital Management Committee approved Mr. Andrews' recommendation that he should be sent on a Clinical Teachers' Course. It is fair to Mr. Harrison to say that he was unhappy at the

decision to leave Mr. Crowson as a charge nurse in Poplars Villa and that he wrote a memorandum to Mr. Andrews, saying that it would probably be in everybody's best interests if he could be moved to a less stressful villa and urging that his future performance be very carefully supervised.

Conclusions

102. We are satisfied that Mr. Crowson told the truth and that Mr. Large assaulted patients HH, CC and DD as described.

103. We were impressed by the manner in which Mr. Crowson gave his evidence. There was no sign of exaggeration. The details of the assaults did not bear any of the hallmarks of a concocted story. We did not consider that Mr. Shrimpton's memory would have been very good even when he was interviewed by the police on 22 February, and we were satisfied that Mr. Crowson told him of the assaults on the afternoon of the day they occurred. In our view no one concocting an untrue story would say the assaults occurred upstairs if the patients were downstairs: neither would he say that one of them occurred in the presence of another member of the staff. None of the assaults was sufficiently serious necessarily, or even probably, to have left marks for Dr. Dutton to have seen when he carried out his examination about 55 hours later.

The Slapping of Patients

104. This is a convenient point at which to consider some other evidence given during this part of our inquiry which throws light on whether other staff from time to time slapped or hit patients.

105. Mr. Crowson distinguished between the assaults on HH and DD and that on CC. He said that the kind of assault that was made on HH and DD seemed to be accepted by some members of the staff: over half of the charge nurses had a very strict attitude and taught their nurses to do things properly, but others accepted some unjustifiable force.

106. Mr. Taylor, a ward orderly in Beech Villa, said that he had slapped the patient Robert Robertson on occasions, and knew that this had been done " at odd times " by other members of the staff. He said that this was done to discourage Robert Robertson from persistently asking for tea. He agreed that a light blow would do no good and that on the four or so occasions he had resorted to this method of control he had given a hard slap on the face. He said that he had only actually seen other members of the staff slap Robert Robertson on " one or two " occasions, and that on those occasions the slaps had been " round the face ". The slaps were given to teach the patient to behave, " to go back and sit down ", and they were " fairly hard ". He could not remember if he had seen this method of control used on other patients, but agreed that in talk amongst the staff it was regarded as unrealistic to control violent patients without slapping them, particularly when there are a number of them together with too few staff.

107. Mr. Davies, the charge nurse, said " I have slapped a patient ". As we understood his evidence a light tap was acceptable, but a " brutal slapping " was not. Mr. Davies tapped the hands of the patients in the low grade room if they stretched out their hands to grab some tea. " By tapping them ", he ex-

plained, " they draw their hand away thereby preventing an accident ". Later the following questions were asked and answers given.

> Q. " What is the object of slapping as opposed to catching hold of his wrist or hand to restrain him? " A. " Time. If you were one side of a table and the patient was the other side and grabbed something, you would not perhaps have time to grab hold of his wrist ".

> Q. " You are meaning you would have time to slap? " A. " As he saw your hand coming he would draw his hand back again ".

> Q. " You mean when he saw your hand coming to catch hold of his wrist he would draw his hand back? " A. " More than likely, yes ".

> Q. " What is wrong in that? You have achieved your object ". A. " There is nothing wrong with that ".

> Q. " Is the purpose of slapping to cause some pain? " A. " No, Sir ".

> Q. " Is the purpose of slapping to some extent to teach him a lesson? " A. " It may be a way of getting through to him that it is wrong to do what he was doing, when you have given him a tap ".

108. At another time Mr. Davies likened the minor slapping which he found acceptable to the chastising he would give his own children. When he was asked whether hospital policy permitted the slapping of patients under any circumstances, he replied " A small slap, I presume it was. Not to mark or bruise. But, as I explained, you would just slap them like you were slapping your own children ".

109. This is in our view an unwise and dangerous attitude towards slapping. It leaves out of account that a violent adult requires a very much harder slap to deter him than a child. It is too easy in circumstances of the kind that prevailed in Beech Villa for slaps on the hand to escalate into slaps on the face, and it will not always stop there. Once some measure of assault, as opposed to physical restraint, is accepted as a legitimate method of training patients it seems to us inevitable that it will be used to control violence by patients.

110. We are satisfied that assaults of the kind witnessed by Mr. Crowson took place more often than Mr. Taylor admitted, and that some of the staff felt that it was unrealistic to expect anything else in an understaffed villa crowded with the hospital's most difficult and violent patients. Some people are less able to control themselves than others. Counselling and help for staff in the light of a clear hospital policy was essential to prevent some members of the staff resorting to violence in such circumstances. This they did not receive, and yet they were carrying the real burden imposed by the policy of overcrowding and underfinancing.

The Death of Robert Robertson

111. Robert Robertson was born in 1931 and was admitted to South Ockendon Hospital in 1956. He was transferred to Beech Villa in 1963. He was subnormal, suffered from epilepsy and had a schizophrenic personality. He was unpredictable in behaviour and frequently attacked staff and other patients. He was often attacked by other patients. On many occasions he threw crockery about. He had a passion for cups of tea and pestered staff for it. If they refused he often became violent.

112. On one occasion he had scratched Mr. Large's face. On another occasion, said Mr. Large, " I went on one morning at 7 o'clock, and he came up and pulled a gold wristwatch off my wrist on an expandable strap and smashed it to smithereens with the heel of his boots ".

113. Robert Robertson died from internal injuries at about 3.15 p.m. on 20 February 1969. The only person who has claimed to see what caused those injuries is Mr. Large. He says that he saw another patient JJ, who has violently assaulted patients on several occasions, stamping on Robert Robertson's stomach. Before we consider the evidence of Mr. Large we propose to set out in chronological order the other events of that day and the following day after the assaults on HH, CC and DD. Where there was any dispute about any material evidence we shall indicate the area of the dispute and make a finding of fact.

   i. At about 7.45–8.00 a.m. Mr. Maghoo, who was looking after the low grade patients in the separate room on the ground floor, saw Mr. Large approaching with Robert Robertson. Mr. Large was pulling him towards the low grade room by the back of his collar. Robert Robertson was trying to go in the opposite direction. Mr. Large managed to pull him into the low grade room but he continued to resist until he slipped. Mr. Large still had hold of his collar and broke his fall. He asked Mr. Maghoo to keep an eye on him as he had been aggressive. He did not tell Mr. Maghoo that JJ had been in a fight with or kicked or stamped on Robert Robertson. He left Robert Robertson sitting on the floor and shortly afterwards he lay down.

   ii. At about 8.30–8.40 a.m. a ward orderly brought the patients' breakfast to the low grade room. He handed a tray with many plates of porridge on it to Mr. Maghoo. As Mr. Maghoo started to take the tray of porridge round the patients Robert Robertson seized the tray and upset all the porridge. Mr. Maghoo then telephoned Mr. Large and told him what had happened and that he could not manage him and asked him to remove him. Mr. Large came and collected him between 8.25 and 8.45 a.m. Mr. Maghoo did not see where he took him.

   iii. Mr. Moothoo, a student nurse, helped Mr. Large to serve the breakfast to the patients in the day room at about 8.30 a.m. While they were doing this Mr. Large told him that Robert Robertson had caused trouble earlier that day. He also recalled that Mr. Large had said something about Robert Robertson being upset or having been hit by another patient.

   iv. Mr. Bass said that when he arrived on duty between 8.00 and 9.00 a.m. Mr. Large had said something to him about having found Robert Robertson lying on the floor. He thought that Mr. Large had said that it was the floor of the low grade room.

   v. At about 9.15 a.m. Mr. Maghoo took the low grade patients to the toilets. In order to get from the day room into the toilets it was necessary to pass through a lobby with a door on either side. Mr. Maghoo found Robert Robertson in this lobby but could not remember whether the door leading into it from the day room was locked. It will be recalled that Dr. Harfst in his letter of 13 January 1969 said that because of the shortage of siderooms " quite often violent patients have to be isolated

28

in a lobby in the lavatory, and this was used as a temporary side room ". Mr. Maghoo was carrying some clean linen, and as he passed Robert Robertson he grabbed some of the linen and " went straight to the toilet and put them in the toilet ". Mr. Maghoo locked himself and the low grade patients into the toilet area leaving Robert Robertson in the lobby. When he left about half an hour later Robert Robertson was still there. He told Mr. Large that Robert Robertson was in the lobby but did not tell him about the linen.

vi. Mr. Moothoo had a tea break which began at 10.00 a.m., or shortly before, and lasted for about 20 minutes. He then returned to the day room and watched the patients. While there he noticed Robert Robertson in the day room close to the door to the toilets. " He was very agitated and very disturbed ". He said " Looking back now, I think he looked quite ill to me, but at that time I had no experience at all ". He was asked " Looking back on it now, with your experience, what was it you saw then which makes you think now that he was looking ill ?" He replied " He was sort of dazed, very pale, and very agitated ". Mr. Moothoo called Mr. Maghoo over to see to Robert Robertson and left them together.

vii. Between 10.45 and 11.00 a.m. Mr. Bass was working in the dormitories when he saw Mr. Large leading Robert Robertson by the hand. " He was in a very weak condition and he looked glassy-eyed and could hardly stand on his legs . . . he was also bleeding from his mouth ". Mr. Large in his evidence described him as " slightly groggy " at that time. We are satisfied that Mr. Bass' language gives a more accurate description of his condition.

viii. Mr. Large then asked Mr. Bass to go to the office with them to assist him to record particulars of Robert Robertson's injuries. Mr. Bass examined him and described the injuries to Mr. Large who stood beside him writing them down on the Injury Report. Mr. Large stated in that report that the injury had occurred at 7.15 a.m., and under the section that required him to record exact details of how and where the injury occurred he wrote " Patient became disturbed in day room and threw plates at other patients, fell over several times and was hit by patient JJ". He recorded the injuries thus. " Graze left side of body 6″ long. 1 bruise centre of spine, 1 bruise below right shoulder blade, 1 bruise forehead ".

ix. After this examination Mr. Bass put Robert Robertson to bed and about 11.30 a.m. Robert Robertson asked him for some water. Mr. Bass continued " I said ' How do you feel? ' He said ' I have a pain in my tummy. I went to the dentist yesterday ' which I presume was the cause of the bleeding from the mouth ". Mr. Large said in evidence that when he took Robert Robertson up to the dormitory he told him that he had a headache. We do not accept that he complained of a headache. In his statement to the police on 21 February 1969 Mr. Large said Robert Robertson had told him "I've got a bit of a tummy ache, I would like to go to bed ".

x. At about 12.00 noon Dr. Jones saw Mr. Large in the pay queue and stopped to talk to him as he had still to visit Beech Villa. Mr. Large said that he had a problem with Robert Robertson. They went to the villa and Mr. Large said that he was very worried about Robert Robertson's mental condition. He said that he had been throwing plates about and had been fighting with JJ, and he was worried that he would get the worst of it in a fight with JJ. Mr. Large never told Dr. Jones anything about Robert Robertson having been kicked or stamped on, but he did say that he was unsteady and swaying on his feet. Dr. Jones said he would take Robert Robertson's drug card and speak to the Chief Pharmacist about the problem and call back later. He signed the injury card without seeing or examining Robert Robertson. He agreed that he should not have done this. Dr. Jones agreed that the reported unsteadiness and swaying could indicate a serious condition, but that this would depend on the cause. He agreed that they could be due to his mental condition or to the effects of his fight and fall, and that an examination was necessary before attributing them to one cause rather than the other. He said that he had concluded that Robert Robertson's mental condition was the cause of his reported unsteadiness and swaying, but he agreed that this was an unwarranted assumption in the absence of any examination. Dr. Jones left the villa between 12.45 and 12.55 taking Robert Robertson's drug card with him.

xi. Mr. Davies took over from Mr. Large just before 1.00 p.m. He was shown the accident report. He did not go straight to Robert Robertson because he believed that he had just been examined by Dr. Jones whom he had seen leaving the villa as he arrived. Mr. Large had recorded in the informal handover book used by charge nurses to pass on information to the charge nurse taking over that JJ had " hit " Robert Robertson.

xii. At about 1.00 p.m. Mr. Taylor went to get his coat before going off duty. He glanced into the patients' toilet and saw Robert Robertson in a semi-conscious condition. He and Mr. Moothoo assisted him back to bed. Neither of them reported what had happened to the charge nurse, Mr. Taylor because he was only a ward orderly, and Mr. Moothoo because he assumed that the patient had been sedated.

xiii. At about 1.10 p.m. Mr. Davies went to the dormitory and found Robert Robertson lying on the floor in a semi-collapsed state. He asked what the matter was and Robert Robertson replied " I feel dizzy ". Having put him on the bed and given Mr. Crowson instructions to treat him for shock Mr. Davies telephoned the nursing administration office who got in touch with Dr. Benton.

xiv. Dr. Benton arrived at the villa at 1.30 p.m. She found that Robert Robertson was unconscious, his abdomen was distended, his heart sounds were very poor, his pulse was 72, and he was very cold. Dr. Benton could not get a blood pressure reading. He was transferred to the Gloucester Clinic where Dr. Harfst saw him at 2.30 p.m. He thought that he might have perforated one of his internal organs and ordered an X-ray. He died on the X-ray table at 3.15 p.m.

xv. On the afternoon of 21 February 1969 Dr. Whitehead carried out a postmortem examination at Thurrock Mortuary. He made the following findings:—

    a. There was a recent bruise and abrasion of the left shoulder about one inch in diameter.

b. There was a recent superficial bruise and abrasion running from the left iliac crest upwards and inwards towards the spine about $7\frac{1}{2}''$ long.

c. There was a small laceration on the back of the scalp.

d. There were no external marks on the abdominal wall, but internal examination revealed longitudinal splitting and perforation in the anterior wall of the transverse colon, and surrounding bruising of the omentum. There was some bruising in the mesocolon of the ascending and descending colon on each side. There was extensive bruising round the duodenum and head of the pancreas and there was bleeding into the mesentery of the small bowel. There was a little peri-renal bruising over the anterior surfaces of the kidneys and bruising round the right suprarenal.

114. Dr. Whitehead expressed the following opinions:—

i. Death was the result of bruising and laceration of the colon and mesentery.

ii. The internal injuries could have been produced if Robert Robertson was lying on the floor with somebody stamping or jumping on him. Alternatively, they could have been caused if he had been forced over a bedrail or ledge of some sort and pressure applied from behind. In either case considerable pressure would have had to be applied even if the stomach muscles were lax. If the muscles were rigid, as might be expected if someone knew he was being attacked, then an even greater degree of force would be required. He thought it would be a painful injury and could not visualise it occurring without severe winding. The length and width of the injuries were consistent with them having been caused by the sole of a shoe.

iii. The $7\frac{1}{2}''$ abrasion was probably caused when Robert Robertson was lying down and could have been caused by the toe of a shoe.

115. Mr. Large told us that he accompanied Mr. Knopp downstairs when he went off duty, at about 7.00 a.m., and then returned to the first floor to quell a disturbance in the dormitory. He then went downstairs again and as he passed the kitchen he saw there were plates and teacups and tea all over the place. There was total confusion. He said he knew that Robert Robertson was responsible because of previous similar conduct, so he went into the day room where " there was all hell let loose ". As he went in he saw JJ through the crowd halfway down the room. " From what I could see at first, I knew he was apparently beating someone. I forced my way through to get towards him, and as I got close I saw [Robert Robertson] going down on the floor. He went down and this chap's legs were going up and down in a stamping motion ". He saw three or four stamps at the most; they landed in the region of the chest and stomach. JJ was wearing leather slippers. Mr. Large said he pulled JJ away to the side of the ward and then attended to Robert Robertson who was on his elbows. He asked him if he was all right and he said he was. " He appeared slightly breathless. He was on about (having a cup of) tea. He was probably suffering from shock, but there was no indication of any severe shock or other severe injury ". He then took him along to Mr. Maghoo in the low grade room.

116. The events that followed have already been set out in paragraphs 113 and 114. Mr. Large said that he did not know why Robert Robertson was in the toilet area.

117. Mr. Large was asked why he had filled in the injury report as he did, and in answer to the question whether he had seen Robert Robertson fall down several times he said " I saw him fall more than once, Sir; yes; on my way towards him through the crowd. How long this had been going on I don't know ".

Q. " You saw him fall down and get up—is that it? " A. " He did not get right up. All I could see was a person up and down quickly. As I got towards him there was obviously a fight going on at the time ".

Q. " Was there a time when he went down and was stamped on? " A. " Yes ".

Q. " Before that time, what was it you had seen as you made your way from the door? " A. " I saw him through the crowd as I approached ".

Q. " What did you see him do that made you write that? " A. " He was rolling. He went from one place to another. I imagine he was trying to get up. He had fallen, or been pushed, but I could not see. I never saw anything until I got in very close proximity to these two patients ".

Q. " Did you see him fall down several times? " A. " As I say, I saw his body going down ".

Q. " Did you see him fall down several times? " A. " He fell on the floor several times; once or twice ".

Q. " You say you imagine he got up. That indicates to me that you did not see him get up?" A. " Well I was not sure. It was such a confused scene. That was the impression it gave me. I might be wrong, but that is the impression I have. I put it down at the time. That was my impression ".

Q. " Forgive me asking you; if all that was so unclear and confused, why not put in the one thing that you say you saw clearly, without any doubt— stamping three or four times? " A. "Well that is the way I interpreted it at the time ".

118. After Mr. Large had completed his examination-in-chief, but before Counsel for the Committee had completed his cross-examination, Mr. Large was admitted to Mabledon Hospital as an inpatient suffering from a depressive illness. The Committee was informed at the beginning of November that it would be a minimum of eight weeks before he would be fit to give evidence and it might be longer. It seemed to us unnecessary to prolong the inquiry or to subject Mr. Large to further questioning.

Conclusions on how Robert Robertson's internal injuries were caused

119. We are satisfied that Mr. Large saw Robert Robertson being aggressive to another patient, probably JJ, between 7.00 and 7.45 a.m. and that it was for this reason he pulled him struggling into the low grade room and told Mr. Maghoo to keep an eye on him as he was being aggressive.

120. We are satisfied that Robert Robertson continued to be obstreperous until about the time he left the lobby leading to the toilet area shortly after 10.00 a.m. We consider it probable that he had been placed in the lobby as a temporary side room.

121. We reject Mr. Large's evidence that he saw JJ stamping on Robert Robertson. Our reasons for rejecting this evidence are:—

    i. Nothing that Mr. Large said or wrote before going off duty referred to his having seen Robert Robertson being jumped or stamped on.

    ii. Mr. Large did not fill in the injury report until after Robert Robertson had gone to bed in an unwell condition at 11.00 a.m. It is in our opinion inconceivable that he would have filled in the injury report as he did if he had seen another patient jumping or stamping on Robert Robertson earlier that day, particularly when that was the only activity which he claims to have seen clearly.

    iii. It is equally inconceivable that he would have failed to describe this jumping or stamping to Dr. Jones later that morning.

    iv. It is highly improbable that Robert Robertson would have been struggling as he was brought to the low grade room if he had immediately before been stamped or jumped upon with sufficient force to cause the internal injuries described by Dr. Whitehead. Mr. Large told Mr. Maghoo that Robert Robertson had been aggressive, and he was still behaving in an aggressive manner as he was brought to the low grade room.

122. We are unable to reach any sure conclusion as to the manner or circumstances in which Robert Robertson received the internal injuries from which he died, and we are satisfied that no other enquiry or proceedings would enable a sure conclusion to be arrived at.

Subsequent History

123. On 3 April 1969 a summons alleging manslaughter of Robert Robertson was served on JJ, and at a Court held at the hospital on 10 April he was committed for trial at Chelmsford Assizes. On 25 April the prosecution were prepared to offer no evidence against JJ, but Mr. Justice Thesiger ruled that a jury should be empanelled to determine whether he was fit to plead to the indictment in support of which the prosecution were not seeking to tender evidence. The jury determined that JJ was unfit to plead to the indictment and the Judge ordered that he should be admitted to such hospital as the Secretary of State should specify. JJ was returned to South Ockendon Hospital.

124. On 16 December 1969 the Court of Criminal Appeal quashed the verdict of the jury on the ground that the trial of issue of whether he was unfit to plead should have been postponed to permit the prosecution to tender no evidence against him. If this had been done he would have been acquitted.

125. On 22 January 1970 JJ again appeared at Chelmsford Assizes, the prosecution offered no evidence against him and he was found not guilty of the manslaughter of Robert Robertson.

126. Towards the end of July 1971 it was learned at the hospital that the police were making further enquiries into the death of Robert Robertson. In April 1972 it was known that the Director of Public Prosecutions had decided not to reopen the matter.

127. In June 1969 Mr. Harrison received an 18–page report of the police investigation. This pointed out that even on his own version of events Mr. Large

had obviously been negligent. Mr. Harrison did not read the report or show it to anyone else. Nobody connected with the hospital considered the question whether Mr. Large's own version of events revealed him as unfit to continue as a charge nurse. The attitude of those at the hospital seems to have been that once an enquiry is handed over to the police the hospital is relieved of any further responsibility in the matter. Nobody seems to have realised that a police investigation of a possible criminal assault is not concerned with departures from an acceptable standard of nursing save insofar as they may assist in determining whether an assault occurred and, if so, who committed it.

128. It was urged before us that it was difficult for the Hospital Management Committee or anyone at the hospital to do anything about any negligent conduct by Mr. Large bearing in mind that JJ's position was not finally resolved until December 1969. We were also asked to remember in this context that following the disciplinary proceedings arising out of the assault on the patient GG, the Group Secretary received a letter from the Ministry of Health dated 14 August 1968 which stated " The Director of Public Prosecutions has in the past expressed the opinion that, where it appears after preliminary enquiries that a criminal offence may have been committed at a hospital, the facts should be reported to the police and no further interrogation of any of the individuals concerned should take place until they have been interviewed by experienced police officers. For this reason, and because charges of a criminal offence are for the Courts to deal with, Hospital Management Committees should not hold disciplinary or other enquiries in such cases until the decision of the police or the Director of Public Prosecutions is known. Action at the hospital should be limited to preliminary enquiries to establish whether there is a *prima facie* case for reporting the matter to the police and, where appropriate, suspending the officer concerned ".

129. We do not accept this argument. From, at the latest, the date of the special court at the hospital on 10 April there was no dispute about the following facts:—

    i. Mr. Large claimed to have seen JJ stamping heavily on Robert Robertson's stomach.

    ii. Internal bruising of that part of his body led to Robert Robertson's death.

    iii. Mr. Large's care of Robert Robertson was inadequate when measured against what he claimed to have seen.

    iv. Mr. Large failed to record in the injury report any reference to Robert Robertson having been stamped on, although at the time the report was made out Robert Robertson was complaining of feeling unwell.

    v. Mr. Large said nothing to Dr. Jones about Robert Robertson having been stamped on.

130. These facts, upon which there was no dispute, revealed clear negligence by Mr. Large, and the Hospital Management Committee should have initiated some action if it had not already been taken by Dr. Dutton and the Nursing Administration. If the Hospital Management Committee were in doubt about the steps they could properly take at that time they should have suspended Mr. Large from duty and consulted the Regional Hospital Board or the Department of Health.

131. Incidents will continue to occur when from a very early stage there is no real doubt that a member of the staff has been negligent, although there is grave doubt as to whether he or another member of the staff or a patient is guilty of an assault. Sometimes the negligence will be by a person who is not suspected of having committed the offence being investigated by the police, although he or she may be a witness.

132. It is in our view important that all Chief Nursing Officers and Hospital Management Committees should remember that the fact that an incident has been referred to the police for criminal investigation in no way absolves them from considering whether the suspect or a witness has fallen below an acceptable standard of nursing care. This will usually involve different issues from those considered by the police in deciding whether a criminal offence has been committed. We believe that incidents of negligence or bad nursing practice may sometimes go unchecked, and even uncommented on, because a matter has been referred to the police for criminal investigation and this distinction in function has not been appreciated.

133. It is clear from a memorandum and a separate report attached thereto dated 28 February 1969 from Dr. Murray of the Regional Hospital Board to Dr. Ramsay that Dr. Dutton and the responsible officers of the Regional Hospital Board knew at that time that Dr. Jones had signed the injury report without examining Robert Robertson. Either Dr. Dutton or Dr. Ramsay should in our view have spoken to Dr. Jones about this failure and taken some steps to see that this did not happen on other occasions. In April Dr. Ramsay made further enquiries about Dr. Jones' failure to examine the patient, but by this time he had taken up an appointment as a Consultant Psychiatrist at another hospital. A memorandum from Dr. Murray to Dr. Ramsay dated 21 April 1969 is expressed in such terms as to suggest that there might be circumstances in which it was permissible for a doctor to sign an injury report without examining the patient to whom it refers. In our opinion a doctor should always examine the injuries referred to in the report before he signs it. On 14 September 1972 Dr. Dutton issued written instructions to all medical staff in the Group that " accident forms etc. should only be signed *after* examining the patient ".

Events Resulting from the Death of Robert Robertson

134. We have already described in paragraphs 11 and 30 to 35 how in the years up to 1968 the policy of overcrowding came to be adopted. In paragraphs 86 to 90 we described how the Medical Advisory Committee's strong warning of January 1969 on the effects of overcrowding was not brought to the notice of the Hospital Management Committee until after the death of Robert Robertson and how Dr. Dutton's letters to Dr. Ramsay had produced no outward response.

135. The death of Robert Robertson convinced Doctor Ramsay that the Board must look more closely into overcrowding, staff morale and staff recruitment at the hospital. At its first meeting after Robert Robertson's death the Board set up a subcommittee under its chairman, Sir Graham Rowlandson, " to consider with the South Ockendon Group Management Committee and report on the difficulties facing the Group in providing a satisfactory service for mentally subnormal patients, particularly at South Ockendon Hospital, and to suggest short term and long term measures to overcome these difficulties ".

136. The Subcommittee produced a 14 page report towards the end of April 1969. We set out some of their conclusions:—

i. " The level of overcrowding . . . is seriously detrimental to the interests of the patients and staff . . . Although admissions to the hospital had been suspended a month before our visit, the situation is one that calls for urgent remedial action ".

ii. During January, February and March 1969 there had been " 28 recorded major injuries to members of the staff in the hospital and 235 injuries caused to patients by other patients ".

iii. The staff ratio was 1:4 compared with 1:3 recommended by the Department of Health, and 1:2·5 considered desirable by the Board.

iv. " Our general conclusion ", on staff, " is that the staff—are giving loyal and dedicated service to the patients, but that they are working under conditions which are grossly unfair to them. The Ministry's memorandum published with HM(65)104 stated that the development of self confidence, self reliance and self respect in patients was all important. In the overcrowded and understaffed ward units at South Ockendon it is impossible for nurses to exercise the necessary degree of control and supervision over the patients to enable even limited progress to be made in this direction. We can readily understand how, in such circumstances, naturally aggressive patients could be involved in incidents and sustain injuries. Although the nursing standard is good, frustration exists among the staff because the conditions under which they work make it difficult, if not impossible in practice, to carry out the nursing procedures inculcated in their training ".

v. Speaking of some of the incidents we have investigated the Subcommittee reported " We are greatly concerned that existing conditions make such incidents possible despite the best efforts of the staff, and we again mention that there are many episodes of attacks by patients on staff which do not become matters of public discussion. It is only by relief of overcrowding and improvements of ward conditions and nurse/patient ratios that the situation can be altered ".

vi. A review of patients at the end of 1967 had shown that 155 patients should be the responsibility of the various Local Health Authorities, but the whole catchment area had residential accommodation for a total of only 50 subnormal people.

vii. " Immediate consideration [must] be given to the possibility of using vacant hospital accommodation elsewhere in the region, providing this is suitable for this type of patient, to which up to 300 suitable patients can be transferred, to relieve overcrowding ".

137. The Board's Subcommittee was not alone in these conclusions. Dr. Brothwood of the Department of Health accompanied the Subcommittee when it visited the hospital and submitted his own report to the Department. On 12 April the Minister of State and Dr. Brothwood visited the hospital and made a report to the Department. On 14 April the Secretary of State for Social Services, in the course of answering a question in the House of Commons, said " On the evidence of the preliminary report, there is grave overcrowding and also grave under-staffing at this hospital. My officer tells me that the staff at South Ockendon, as at other hospitals for subnormals, are struggling against

unfair odds. Only after a reduction in the number of patients can they hope to provide a satisfactory standard of care ". In the course of answering a supplementary question the Secretary of State said " It is my view, as a result of our first report, that nothing less than a reduction in the number of patients at the hospital will really relieve the situation, and I am consulting with the Board about the possibility of so doing. Until one has done that, as I said in my main answer, a satisfactory standard of care is impossible at this hospital ".

138. In June 1969 the Post Ely Policy Working Party reported that the Group as a whole was 25% overcrowded. " In some wards . . . the degree of overcrowding is tolerable, but in some wards, such as the Poplars and the Beeches, it is quite intolerable and dangerous in degree. Among the effects of the overcrowding are these:—

    a. There are so many patients that the staff cannot adequately attend even to the basic needs of the patients although they spend all their time doing just this.

    b. The existing facilities are not sufficient for the number of patients and not always suited to the type of occupant.

    c. The patients are, therefore, more difficult to keep clean and so are the wards.

    d. Because of the overcrowded conditions, and the fact that patients' wants cannot be fully attended to, their behaviour is much more difficult and, in some cases, dangerous ".

139. The Secretary of State in no way modified his opinion expressed on 14 April 1969. Almost a year later on 23 March 1970 he said in the House of Commons " During recent months I have been seriously concerned by the appalling problems of overcrowding at South Ockendon where a huge mental handicap hospital in the middle of Essex serves a catchment area of $1\frac{1}{2}$ million people in no fewer than ten London Local Authorities. The proper solution for this problem would be for those Local Authorities to provide hostels and halfway houses for a large number of South Ockendon patients, but this is almost impossible to organize with the multiplicity of conflicting authorities. We try to alleviate the trouble but South Ockendon remains dangerously overcrowded ".

140. After the passing of yet another year the Hospital Advisory Service reported in March 1971 " It is obvious that this hospital has been labouring under very great difficulties for a long time. The combination of overcrowding, staff shortages and inadequate provision for the occupation and training of patients give rise to a grave and undeniably dangerous situation. I consider that, while conditions remain as they are, the patients at this hospital remain at risk. There is a limit to the amount of stress which staff on high dependency wards can endure over a prolonged period. Moreover, there is no doubt that patients admitted to some areas within the hospital in the prevailing circumstances could only deteriorate ".

141. These assessments of the position at South Ockendon Hospital between April 1969 and April 1971 all say the same thing in different words. We agree with them. They demand an answer to the following questions:—

Why was the position not appreciated by the Board before the death of Robert Robertson?

Why was the degree of overcrowding still such that it was properly described as dangerous in March 1971, nearly two years after the danger had been appreciated by the Board and the Department?

Why was the position not appreciated by the Board before the death of Robert Robertson?

142. We investigated this with Professor Ramsay upon whose advice the Board depended. He agreed that statistically there was no significant difference in the degree of overcrowding and understaffing between 1965 and 1969. He said that Dr. Dutton and Dr. Matheson, his predecessor as Physician Superintendent, were continuously advising him that the degree of overcrowding and understaffing was " critical ", and that on some occasions the word " dangerous " was used. In spite of these repeated warnings Professor Ramsay considered until after the death of Robert Robertson that there was an acceptable level of overcrowding and an acceptable standard of care. Why? We try to summarise his reasons and make our comments on them below.

    i. Statistics showed that the level of overcrowding did not exceed the national average.

    Comment. In our view Dr. Ramsay concluded from this statistical information that the standard of care must also accord with the national average and therefore be acceptable. In doing so he left out of account the fact that South Ockendon Hospital had a high proportion of severely handicapped patients. Since 1966 Dr. Dutton had restricted admissions to patients who clearly needed hospital treatment. It should have been realised that this would increase the burden on the already overstretched staff. Mr. Huws Jones, a member of the Board, described this trend as the " silting up " process. For example, in 1965 there were 215 patients in wheelchairs and 270 patients with epilepsy. By 1969 those figures had risen to 340 and 310 respectively.

    ii. Consultants in every field were using the word " dangerous ". Some were saying that their operating theatres were dangerous, others that their resources were dangerously inadequate. " This was one of many dangerous situations that one had to face, and one had to weigh the relative danger of the different situations against the amount of capital which was available to remedy the defects. It was a matter of priorities all the time, continuously ". Later in his evidence Professor Ramsay said that, if more money had been spent at South Ockendon Hospital, people would have died elsewhere in the region for lack of maternity departments or modern casualty departments.

    Comment. We accept that Dr. Ramsay was faced with a multitude of demands all of which could not be met. Because there were so many situations being described as dangerous, and not enough money to go round, there was an understandable tendency not to investigate each allegedly dangerous situation as fully as it should have been investigated. The absence of a maternity unit could result in unnecessary deaths, whereas patients at South Ockendon would continue to exist without the improvements being sought.

    iii. Public attitudes and expectations were changing in 1968 and 1969 which led everyone to realise that standards they had accepted in the past " were just not good enough ".

Comment. This argument overlooks paragraphs 14 to 18 of the Ministry of Health Memorandum HM(65)104 " Improving the Effectiveness of the Hospital Service for the Mentally Subnormal " which was sent to all Boards and Management Committees in December 1965. It is perhaps fair to Professor Ramsay that we should state at this point that even in November 1972 the Management Committee members were unable to accept the use of the word " dangerous " as apt to describe the situation in the hospital at any time. We consider their attitude to the Hospital Advisory Service Report's use of the word in a later section of this report (see paragraphs 502 to 516).

iv. Until the issue of HM(69)59 in July 1969 the Board did not regard itself as having " a day to day monitoring responsibility ". It dealt with complaints that reached it but did not take the initiative itself in checking standards. (for comments, see paragraphs 209 to 211).

Why was the degree of overcrowding still such that it was properly described as dangerous by the Hospital Advisory Service in March of 1971 ?

143. In March 1969 the Hospital Management Committee with the approval of the Board banned all admissions to South Ockendon Hospital. This drastic action was supported by the Secretary of State.

144. The Board's officers examined all hospital accommodation in the Region which was vacant or due to be vacated in order to see whether it was suitable to be used or converted for use by mentally handicapped patients. All were unsuitable in construction and incapable of conversion without disproportionately high expenditure except for the Annexe of the London Hospital at Brentwood. This was converted to take 100 mentally handicapped patients at a cost of over £100,000 which came from the Board's capital building allocation. It is now known as Little High Wood and its first patients were admitted on 28 January 1971. It has relieved the overcrowding at South Ockendon by taking 50 of its patients.

145. Having failed to find any other building suitable for conversion the Board produced a crash action programme to deal with the overcrowding, which was sent to the Department at the end of May 1969. Its proposals were:

i. That a new hospital of 550 beds for subnormal patients should be built at Claybury Hospital. It was appreciated that the provision of a hospital of this size on the same site as an existing hospital might not accord with current thinking, but the following considerations seemed important to the Board:

a. This was the revival of a scheme which had originally been included in the 1962 programme but had not been proceeded with because of lack of finance:

b. It was known that a hospital of this size broken down into small " family units " was being built at Northampton with the approval of the Department. Plans were obtained from the Oxford Regional Hospital Board and, after full consultation, the Board were satisfied that they could be used to provide an independent unit at Claybury Hospital with the minimum of delay. It was thought that the cost

39

would be in the region of £2.81 million and that work could start in 1970/71.

    c. No other solution would provide a speedy relief of overcrowding in the Region.

  ii. That while the new hospital was being built four prefabricated units should be built at South Ockendon to relieve overcrowding and permit the upgrading of existing villas. It was estimated that the prefabricated buildings would cost in total about £245,000 and that two of them could be brought into use within six months. The other two would be ready for use within twelve months. It was emphasised that these units would not be used to increase the number of patients in the hospital.

146. These proposals were discussed by the Secretary of State, the Minister of State, Sir Graham Rowlandson, Dr. Ramsay and Mr. Phipps on 30 June 1969. The Secretary of State and his advisers would not approve the proposal for the new hospital at Claybury because it would add to a hospital complex that was already too large. The proposal for the four prefabricated units was also rejected on the ground that, whatever the intention of the Board, the pressure for admission would inevitably lead to a further increase in the number of patients in the hospital.

147. It is unnecessary for us to follow through in this report the talking and the letter-writing that followed the rejection of the Board's proposals. Nothing suggested by the Department solved the problem of how to bring speedy relief to the dangerous degree of overcrowding. The letters and minutes of meetings made a sad and strong contrast to the language in the House of Commons and the reports of the Board's Subcommittee, the Post Ely Policy Working Party and the Hospital Advisory Service. In September 1969 the Department agreed to provide a prefabricated unit to be used in conjunction with Larches Villa. Together they provided accommodation for patients while existing villas were upgraded. But the upgraded villas would contain fewer patients and exacerbate the overcrowding elsewhere.

148. Between February 1969 and February 1970 the number of patients in the hospital was reduced by about 35. From the beginning of that year the Board was under increasing pressure from the Secretary of State to resume admissions to the hospital although he was " seriously concerned by the appalling problems of overcrowding ". Eventually, at the end of July 1970, the Board with the approval of the Hospital Management Committee and consultants, agreed to admit one new patient for every four discharged.

149. We recognise that the pressure from the community to resume admissions was very great and that so long as the ban remained in force there would be families who would suffer great hardship. We recognise that the money which was allocated to the Secretary of State was far less than he hoped for and far less than was urgently needed. So long as the finance available is so far short of reasonable aspiration these acute and painful dilemmas will continue.

150. Between February 1970 and March 1971 the number of patients was reduced by a further 50, most of whom had gone to Little High Wood. This was a reduction of 85 in the two years following the setting up of the Board's Sub-committee. The efforts to reduce numbers received a set back from the decision

to accept a number of short-term admissions to help hard-pressed families. 23 of those admitted for short-term relief could not be returned to their families and so increased the permanent population of the hospital.

151. We report on the reduction of overcrowding since March 1971 in paragraphs 596 to 599.

Allegation of Mr. Hill

152. Mr. Hill was employed as carpenter's mate by a contractor who built side rooms in Beech Villa early in 1970. He told us that, one afternoon, he saw a patient who was lying in bed being struck by a male nurse with a banana which was then fed to the patient without being skinned. He said that he and the carpenter " had a laugh and a joke about it afterwards because only recently have I felt bad about this ". He claimed that he got someone to write down a complaint for him about two days after the incident and that he signed it and put it in the complaints box in the office but heard nothing from the hospital.

153. No trace could be found at the hospital of any such complaint. Mr. Nelson, the carpenter, was unable to recall any incident of the type described and said that he had never seen any ill-treatment of patients in the course of his work. We were not satisfied as to the truth of Mr. Hill's allegations.

Beech Today

154. We visited this villa on three occasions. It is the home of 40 severely disturbed male patients many of whom are very destructive. We were told, and found on two of our visits, that the outer doors were kept locked and that freedom of movement was permitted inside. On our third visit the outer doors were unlocked but the door from the corridor into the large day room was locked, as was the door leading from the day room into the bowl room and thence to the second staircase. The doors into the two smaller day rooms may have been locked at the time of our third visit as all the patients except the low grade patients, who had already gone to bed, were in the large day room. Some were watching television but most were milling about the room in a noisy aimless manner. Their clothes were ill-fitting and some had bare feet. Some efforts have been made to give the villa a homely appearance but it remains a grim institutional building in poor decorative condition with only basic furniture. There are sufficient wardrobes or lockers for the majority of the patients but examination showed that only a tiny proportion were used to store anything.

155. The problems were described to us by Mr. Harding, the Charge Nurse. He came to the hospital as a student nurse in 1949 and has been there ever since. He was appointed to Beech in December 1971. There were then 49 patients. In May 1972 nine of the patients were transferred to Leytonstone House.

156. The average nursing staff on duty by day are a charge nurse and three others. There are three domestic staff who leave by 3.00 p.m., one domestic worker comes in from 5.00 p.m. to 8.00 p.m. to clean the day room and the kitchen and do the washing-up after tea. At the time of our third visit there was one charge nurse, three students, two nursing assistants and one domestic worker.

41

157. Mr. Harding introduced group training programmes to improve eating habits and reduce incontinence. He said that the eating habits of most of the patients have greatly improved, and that the number using knives, forks and spoons has increased from three to about twelve. He told us that the amount of incontinence has been reduced by up to 50% by ensuring regular visits to and use of the lavatories.

158. Mr. Harding was insistent that the urgent need was a further reduction in the number of patients. Ideally he would like to see the number reduced to 20. He did not consider that an increase of staff with the present number of patients would be of much help as there is not sufficient accommodation to permit more group training programmes and group activities.

159. The lockers cannot be used at present because the patients remove articles from them and throw them about the rooms or out of the windows. Behaviour modification training is essential before any real benefit can be derived by the patients from their presence. Until that time the lockers and wardrobes are only of ornamental and statistical value.

160. Mr. Harding felt that the introduction of personal clothing would create a great amount of extra work for staff until the behaviour of the patients has improved.

Conclusions

161. This villa has reached the 1969 interim standard for the amount of floor space per patient, but this in our view is not an acceptable standard for this type of patient in this kind of building. Urgent steps must be taken to reduce the number of patients by at least ten.

CHAPTER V

CYPRESS VILLA

162. In March 1967 the first patients entered Cypress Villa. It was a specially built medium security unit to serve the whole Region. It ceased to be a security unit for the region in December 1969 as a result of the vociferous, often unbridled, but always justified complaints of the mother of one of its patients. Thereafter it continued as a security unit, in fact if not in name, serving the needs of the hospital.

163. These events form a convenient framework in which to examine the administrative side of care and the problems created by the clinical autonomy of consultants at South Ockendon Hospital. We propose therefore to consider them in eight sections:

  i. The planning of the villa as a security unit and its operation until September 1967.
  ii. The changes introduced by Dr. Harfst on his arrival in September 1967.
  iii. The effect of clinical autonomy.
  iv. Patient S.
  v. 1969–72 Cypress Villa as a ward for disturbed patients.
  vi. John Meter.
  vii. Allegations of violence in 1972.
  viii. Cypress Villa today.

Planning and Operation up to September 1967

164. The Report of the Working Party on Special Hospitals (February 1961) identified the problem of patients in psychiatpic hospitals who, while not requiring the degree of security provided in Special Hospitals, were difficult more or less continuously and could not be satisfactorily contained in all hospitals. The Working Party therefore recommended (paragraph 27) that " security arrangements short of those provided at Special Hospitals should continue to be provided in the National Health Service, and that, with this in mind, Regional Hospital Boards should arrange their psychiatric services so as to ensure that there is a variety of types of hospital unit, including some secure units and that transfers can be made between them as necessary ". The Working Party did not give any guidance as to how the secure units might be organised or run. Neither did HM (61) 69 which was issued in July 1961 to give advice to hospital authorities on how this recommendation of the Working Party should be implemented.

165. Very much more help was given by a memorandum sent out by the Ministry of Health to the Secretaries of all Regional Hospital Boards on 22 November 1961. Paragraph 5 of the memorandum included this guidance. " What form the units will take will depend on various factors, in particular the number of such patients and the staffing situation. For example, it might merely be necessary to provide a locked ward or wards at a hospital where the staffing

situation was good enough to allow the close supervision of the patients needing security while they were using the recreational or occupational facilities, presumably together with the other patients in the hospital. Often, however, it may be preferable to have a separate security unit with its own provision for occupation and recreation. Such a unit is of course not intended to provide the kind of security of the Special Hospitals, nor to deal with persistently dangerous or violent patients. Its main object is to make it difficult for patients to walk out at will—though even a prison cannot guarantee that there will never be escapes. The main needs seem to be locked doors, windows that cannot be too easily got through, and a barrier round the perimeter which, while not unclimbable, will present some obstacle. It is, however, difficult to be precise about the physical requirements of a security unit because they are so much affected by the degree of supervision which can be provided and by the realisation on the part of the staff that they are concerned with patients for whom security is an important part of treatment ".

166. On 18 June 1962 the Ministry of Health sent a letter to all Regional Hospital Boards asking what secure accommodation was then in existence and what was proposed.

167. Professor Ramsay who was then Deputy Senior Administrative Medical Officer had delegated to him the responsibility for the capital programme of the Board. As part of this delegated duty he had to advise the Board whether there should be a security unit, where it should be placed and what its nature should be. He consulted the Board's Psychiatric Advisory Committee who advised in September 1963 that there should be a unit at South Ockendon Hospital similar to that at Little Plumstead Hospital.

168. The Hospital Management Committee were against the proposal unless they received assurances that the substantial capital cost would not affect the money they so badly needed to provide more housing and better facilities for staff. At a meeting of Board and Hospital representatives on 24 January 1964 Dr. Dutton said that if a security unit was provided it was also necessary to provide a psychology department. Without it, he said, patients " would simply become prisoners in the unit with little hope of improvement or discharge ". The Board supported these views and wrote fully to the Ministry of Health on 5 February 1964 asking for extra finance to carry out the building of the unit and the provision of the psychology department. The Ministry of Health finally wrote on 24 June 1964 that no additional funds could be made available but added " considerable importance is attached to the provision of security accommodation and it is hoped that the Board will be able to proceed with this project as soon as possible ".

169. So plans proceeded for the erection of the security unit without the psychology department. Professor Ramsay told us that the building was planned in the belief that " patients would be able to enjoy the use of other facilities in the hospital such as occupational therapy and physiotherapy in controlled circumstances ".

170. During the building of the security unit Dr. Dutton, Mr. Whiting (a Management Committee member) and Mr. Hubbard (the Chief Male Nurse) visited the security unit at Little Plumstead Hospital. Mr. Hubbard wrote a report in which he summarised their conclusions thus:—" It was noted that

although we were assured that the South Ockendon Hospital project closely resembled the female security unit at Little Plumstead, there are in fact variations in structure to such a degree that the whole appearance has undergone a considerable change. The units at Little Plumstead, whilst being suited to their function, are so built that their true purpose is not obvious on inspection from the outside ". Professor Ramsay told us that when he visited Cypress in 1968 " It looked like a prison. . . . The windows are small. The unit had lost in the translation by the architect something of the appearance of the former unit. It did not look the sort of unit I would have wished to be in one of the Board's hospitals ".

171. When the unit opened in March 1967 the Board were still looking for a consultant with suitable experience to be responsible for it. Until one could be found Dr. Dutton assumed responsibility. He received no guidance from the Board or its officers as to how he should set about the job or what type of patient he should admit. He was very selective in those he admitted, " I was trying to choose patients, I must admit, who would present the least problems to a new unit where the staff were untrained in security and I myself had never worked in a special hospital. One was selective and tried to choose those who would fit into a developing unit ".

172. During the time that Dr. Dutton was responsible for Cypress there were never more than seven patients in the villa, and it is clear from an examination of the ward report books that the majority of them were going to the workshop daily and that there were regular visits by most of the patients to dances and cinema shows. It is clear from notes written by Dr. Dutton for the guidance of charge nurses, in March, that he was determined that the villa was not just a " medical prison ", " the outlook must be progressive and therapeutic ". He emphasised that there must be " firm, rational but always reasonable discipline ".

173. In April Mr. Hubbard instructed the staff on the villa that seclusion could only be applied with the permission of the Medical Officer in Charge, that it could only be applied for thirty minutes after which the door must be unlocked for at least thirty minutes and that there must be a nurse outside the room at all times when a patient was secluded in it.

174. In July 1967 Dr. Dutton varied these instructions and said that patients might be put in the side rooms for therapeutic reasons, but that the doctor must be informed immediately afterwards. At the same time he said that patients were to be in the villa for two weeks before being allowed out to take part in outside activities, that industrial work was to be provided in the villa for those patients who could not leave it, and that normally hospital clothing should be worn and private clothing kept for visiting. He told us " We have awful problems with private clothing, keeping tracks of it, and one tries to keep their own private, more respectable clothing, if that is the right word, for privileged occasions; so rather than let them use their own clothes and have them destroyed on the ward we felt that if we gave them hospital clothing they could then have their best clothing as a privilege for good behaviour. This is part of the system of earning privileges ". We do not agree. We regard this ruling on private clothing as no more than an effort to present a respectable argument to eliminate the undoubted administrative inconveniences created by the wearing of personal clothing. The slow build-up of patients in a new villa was an admirable occasion

for Dr. Dutton to have carried out the Departmental policy that clothing for long-stay patients should be personally owned and that if it was supplied by the hospital it should be on a personal basis. The wearing of personal clothes would have done something to overcome the prison-like atmosphere created by the building. We are satisfied that the inconvenience of personal clothing was pointed out to Dr. Dutton by the staff and that he followed the line of least resistance.

175. Dr. Dutton said that new patients were kept in side rooms for about two days but that apart from that there was virtually no seclusion while he was in charge of Cypress. A study of the ward report book supports his recollection which we accept.

176. We cannot, however, agree that any patient admitted to a locked ward need spend his first days in a side room unless he arrives in a disturbed state. Such seclusion makes assessment more difficult and postpones integration. Subject to this criticism and his instructions on the wearing of private clothes, Dr. Dutton on the whole ran Cypress as in our view it should have been run. He was sensible in choosing the patients carefully, and we feel that he was assisted by his dislike of the whole concept of a security unit. He should have urged this cautious approach on Dr. Harfst when he became the consultant responsible.

Changes Introduced by Dr. Harfst

177. Dr. Harfst arrived at South Ockendon towards the end of September 1967. It was his first consultant post. He had qualified in general medicine nine years before. He had had no psychiatric experience until about 1962 when he became a junior member of the psychiatric staff of an ordinary psychiatric hospital in Scotland. He spent $3\frac{1}{2}$ years in this position during which he attended post-graduate courses and qualified in psychiatry, winning a gold medal. He then spent a year as an assistant medical officer at the State Hospital in Carstairs. Dr. Harfst said that the regime in that hospital was more strict than in the Special Hospitals in England.

178. The Regional Hospital Board had been searching for about nine months for a consultant to join the staff at South Ockendon Hospital with particular responsibility for running the security unit. A factor in choosing Dr. Harfst was undoubtedly his experience of security at Carstairs. The job description stated " South Ockendon Hospital contains a modern, well-equipped clinical unit. There will shortly be opened a new unit for the treatment of male subnormal psychopaths under conditions of security. This will be run on therapeutic lines and the consultant appointed will be expected to participate actively in the dynamic approach to the treatment of this class of patient ". The relationship of the consultant to the Physician Superintendent was described thus: " although the officer appointed will have full consultant (clinical) responsibility the Physician Superintendent is broadly responsible for and answerable directly to the Hospital Management Committee for all matters concerning the maintenance of the medical service and the overall medical administration of the South Ockendon Group ".

179. Dr. Harfst was given no indication by the Board or its officers as to how they interpreted the words " under conditions of security ". Professor Ramsay said that if Dr. Harfst had asked for guidance it would have been given. He explained " It has not been the normal policy for my office and the Board to

write a detailed operational policy on the clinical care of patients. When the Board appoints a consultant they do so in the knowledge that he is a man chosen by a professional committee who is an expert in his particular field. He is more expert than the Senior Administrative Medical Officer or the Board. It is for him to determine his operational policy within his own professional knowledge and within the resources of the unit of which he has charge ".

180. This was a new kind of unit for the Board and one of which Dr. Harfst had no previous experience. The job description gave no effective guidance. It was in our opinion the responsibility of the Board to give greater guidance on policy than it did. Dr. Harfst should at least have been told that it was intended that patients should make use of the general hospital facilities such as occupational and industrial therapy and physiotherapy.

181. The reluctance to give greater guidance in our view stemmed from too great a regard for, and an unimaginative approach to, what may be called the doctrine of the clinical autonomy of the consultant. As will be seen subservience to this doctrine was too often permitted to become a substitute for much needed action and worked to the disadvantage of patients rather than their benefit.

182. Dr. Harfst commenced work at South Ockendon Hospital on 25 September 1967. He had a very heavy work load. In addition to responsibility for the development of Cypress, which then contained seven patients, he was responsible for another ten villas including Beech. He did outpatient work and was responsible for advising two London Boroughs on subnormality services. He had to deal with all the forensic work of the hospital, including visits to prisons, remand centres, borstals, approved schools and other hospitals. He was Honorary Secretary to the Medical Advisory Committee, and Control Infection Officer for the Group. Dr. Harfst also acted as representative of the Group on the North-East Metropolitan Regional Hospital Medical Services Committee of the British Medical Association.

183. Examination of the ward report books for Cypress shows that the arrival of Dr. Harfst was followed by an immediate and striking change of policy. On 27 September it was recorded that a patient who exposed himself indecently to a young lady while returning from the workshop was to be put to bed in a side room for at least three days. He was allowed to get up on 1 October and permitted some exercise in the afternoon. He was released from the side room on the following day. On 17 October WW, a patient who was often in trouble, was found with another patient using a cigarette lighter. Patient WW's medical records show that he was also alleged to have been abusive and threatening. Both patients were put into side rooms where they remained until 24 October although they were well behaved during that time. On 29 October Patient WW was again in trouble for difficult but not violent behaviour and was confined to a side room. The ward report book shows that he was allowed up for the first time on 6 November. These are only samples of the manner in which side rooms began to be used.

184. The second major change during the month following Dr. Harfst's appointment was that patients were no longer taken out of the villa for occupational or industrial therapy or for dances and cinema shows. Instead of being the reasonably liberal but firmly disciplined security villa it had been under Dr. Dutton, with the patient using the general facilities of the hospital whenever

possible, it became a tightly closed regime using side rooms in a punitive manner. Dr. Harfst made no secret of what he was doing and we shall consider at a later stage why these changes were allowed to take place without check and virtually without comment. First we set out why the changes occurred.

185. Dr. Harfst said that when he arrived at South Ockendon he found that the staff at all levels were extremely anxious about and hostile towards Cypress. There had recently been a sexual assault by a patient from another villa on a child who lived nearby, and staff felt that the patients in Cypress increased the risk of this kind of incident. Moreover there were some staff houses very close to Cypress. In a written statement to the Committee which formed part of his evidence Dr. Harfst said " My first urgent assessment on arrival was that the staff had considerable cause for anxiety. Several of the patients seemed in my view potentially a great danger and existing levels of staff numbers and expertise were low. . . . I felt that I could not run the unit, at any rate at the beginning, on its existing open lines. My own first admission to the unit which followed very soon also caused further great anxieties to nursing staff and subsequently to myself. The initial decision to run the unit as a closed one was not taken by me with any theoretical viewpoint in mind but rather as it seemed a temporary necessity until further needs became clear ".

186. Dr. Harfst developed this in his oral evidence. " One of the big problems, it seemed to me in discussion with the nursing staff, was that I came with the philosophy of a special hospital which was quite different, foreign and unknown to the nursing staff here. I accepted standards and ways of going about things which I think they were not able to because of their different background. Similarly, my experience of large subnormality hospitals was limited, and, equally, I was not able terribly well to understand them. I was very worried about the nursing staffs' ability to manage acute problems of disturbance in the wards and for this reason I rigidified things, I think, too much; but it was out of fear of injury to staff and staff getting into difficulties ". Later in his evidence he explained this still further:—" all the angles which I thought of with regard to security had to be discussed with staff and had to be translated into some practical terms whilst they had to be done in agreement with them and decisions had to be made through their eyes. I think for this reason in particular I erred too much on the side of security and the system became too rigid ".

187. Dr. Harfst's difficulty in bridging the gap between his short experience of a state hospital in Scotland and the more liberal approach of a large subnormality hospital in England clearly emerges from these passages. He said he was " not able terribly well to understand " the staff. We accept that in an endeavour to understand them better and to give them confidence in the unit and himself he did permit himself to some extent to become a prisoner of his staff's lack of knowledge and natural fears. Nevertheless this is only part of the explanation for the change of policy, for there can be no doubt that Dr. Harfst initiated many changes with an enthusiasm for an extremely high degree of security which was almost obsessional in its intensity.

188. On 13 October 1967 Dr. Harfst prepared a seven-page memorandum containing 24 proposals for making Cypress structurally more secure. The following criticisms and suggestions were included.

i. The front door should be replaced by two doors one behind the other. " The outer door should be solid, heavy and reinforced ".

ii. The winding gear of the windows could be torn off and used as a weapon and a window could be opened sufficiently wide for a man to climb out. A bar to fill the space was not the answer as it was in itself a severe security risk and could also be used as a suspension point from which a patient could hang himself. The only way of managing patients in any of the rooms in the building was for each window to be permanently closed by riveting. This applied also to windows opening on to the central courtyard, as persons from outside might cross the roof in order to liberate the patients inside.

iii. There were too many projections from the floors and walls of the day lavatory which obstructed a clear view of the patients using it.

iv. The ornamental wall by the front door was a severe security risk as it gave access to the roof which as a potential means of access for forceful entry. " Friends and relatives of the patients or even complete strangers may attempt this. It must be remembered that such people will have access to tools, may themselves be expert and experienced housebreakers, and most important may attack the building with force of numbers ".

v. " A night station should be constructed for use of night staff observing the dormitories. It should be a strongly reinforced ' cell ' and should be lockable ".

vi. " In the event of a riot occurring in the building (which is the most dangerous single hazard to be faced by the staff in a community of this kind), as the building stands at present, the staff could quickly be overcome and the building reduced to ruins in a very short space of time ".

189. A bare list of Dr. Harfst's recommendations was submitted to and approved by the Land and Works Sub-Committee. It was not explained that any change of policy was involved.

190. In February 1968 Dr. Harfst produced five pages of " Rules for the Guidance of Night Staff " which were stuck up on a wall of the office. They included:

i. "Patients using the day lavatory should be locked in and observed constantly."

ii. " A patient in a side room who has attracted the attention of a nurse should have his request made clear by conversation through the door. If possible his requirements should be diverted or otherwise met without the door being unlocked or opened ".

iii. " It is exceedingly dangerous to enter a dormitory at night once the patients have been locked in it. Beware of patients trying to inveigle you into unlocking the dormitory door by supplying you with plausible excuses. Try and deal with such patients by talking to them through the door but *never* open it. . . . Beware of diversions (pseudo emergencies created by patients to divert and tie down nursing staff, to assist a mass escape plan) ".

iv. " Never enter a lavatory with only one patient in it for fear of accusation of homosexual assault. . . . Do not enter a side room with a patient in it if you are alone and unobserved for the same reason ".

192. In the eighteen months that followed, the use of side rooms for punitive purposes increased. We give a few more examples from the ward report books.

   i. In February 1968 Patient WW spent another nine days in bed in a side room before being allowed up because he was insolent and threatening towards the staff. Paragraphs 565 to 568 relate the circumstances in which Patient WW spent further time in a side room after making a complaint about a charge nurse.

   ii. On 9 March 1968 a patient was abusive to a nurse and was put in a side room for one day. On the following day he was seen by Dr. Harfst who said that he was to remain there until further notice. He was allowed up nearly four weeks later on 4 April 1968.

   iii. On 8 August 1968 a patient was put in a side room for insolence. He was released on 15 August.

   iv. On 9 October 1968 a patient was put in a side room for being unco-operative and refusing to do what he was asked. He was allowed up eleven days later on 20 October.

192. Every patient who was admitted to Cypress was confined in a side room and deprived of all reasonable comforts. When Dr. Harfst commenced his evidence before us he said that the average time spent by each patient in a side room on admission was three days. He returned after the weekend and said that he had carried out a check and found that the average length of stay in a side room on admission was seven days. " I cannot remember whether I was aware of that at the time, but I think I was not, and I would not be in agreement with it ". He was asked " Would that be too long? " and replied " I would have thought so. I accept responsibility that it occurred, . . . it would be unnecessary, and I think it must have arisen from the nursing staff misunderstanding my views and attitude, and lack of communication; for that I must take responsibility ". In our view Dr. Harfst should have known that most patients were spending more than three days in a side room on admission.

193. The conditions of life in side rooms were completely lacking in dignity and incapable of justification. We summarise the worst features thus.

   i. Although at one time there were beds in the side rooms there came a time when there was only a mattress and a blanket on the floor with no furniture of any kind. Dr. Harfst was asked " Was there any reason for just a mattress on the floor? " He replied " Well, yes. This policy of having beds on the floor in side rooms was a result of discussions I had with the nursing staff who were very keen not to have bedsteads. I would rather myself have had bedsteads but we have had some difficulty in side rooms with patients dismantling bedsteads. On one occasion one patient stood on his bedstead and interfered with lighting apparatus on the ceiling of the room. On another occasion a patient climbed through the ceiling into the roof space. I found that the nursing staff were never very keen on having removable bedsteads in single rooms. What I would personally have liked would have been a fixed bedstead or bed platform, a low platform raising the bed a little off the ground, or, alternatively, what I noticed was fairly usual practice in purpose-built security units is to have a fixed concrete plinth very low on the ground with a mattress on top of it ". The fact that some patients may misuse a bed is no justification for withdrawing beds from all patients in side rooms. So far as we know Dr. Harfst never asked for a fixed bedstead or platform. Dr. Harfst was asked why no other furniture was provided and he said " The only other furniture there would have been alongside the patient's bed would have been a locker, and lockers were not put in the side rooms . . . because we feared that it would be used as a security risk to be destroyed and thrown at staff, and a patient on his first three days in a ward would not be in possession of much ".

ii. The provision of a locker and a chair, which was apparently not considered by Dr. Harfst, would at least have permitted a patient to eat his meals in some comfort. As things were he had to eat his meals sitting on the mattress on the floor without the aid of a knife and fork which were not allowed for fear that they would be used aggressively or in suicide attempts. Once again this rule applied to every new patient, even though he had no history which would lead to a justifiable fear of aggression or attempts at suicide.

iii All a patient's belongings were taken from him on admission. If he asked to be given back his spectacles or pen or pencil or a handkerchief these should have been given to him. Reading matter, even a patient's own, was not provided in a side room unless he asked for it.

iv. Patients were clothed only in pyjamas. If they stood up they had to hold their trousers up with their hands as the cords had been removed so that they could not be used in suicide attempts, whether or not there was any justifiable fear of such an attempt. If a patient had a visitor he was permitted to dress, but after the visit he would have to put his pyjamas on again. Dr. Harfst was asked why patients were dressed for visits. He said " It makes the whole thing pleasanter and more comfortable ".

Q. " Does it mean there is really no medical or psychiatric reason why they should not be in their clothes during the day? " A. " I think it is really simply a matter of nursing tradition . . . ".

Q. " Was there a tradition that those confined to side rooms should be deprived of their clothing? " A. " It was the usual thing ".

Q. " A routine which one had accepted? " A. " Yes . . . ".

Q. " Just to follow that a little further, you have told us that you laid down the regime in Cypress Ward. When did the routine that a patient who was in a side room should be in pyjamas and not in his clothes come into the regime? " A. " Well, I think right from the beginning. I think it was understood by the nursing staff ".

Q. " And by you? " A. " Yes ".

v. Patients had no footwear or dressing gown in the side rooms. These were kept outside for them if they wished to go to the lavatory. They then had to knock on the door for the staff as none of the side rooms could be opened from the inside, even if they were not locked on the outside.

196. In February 1969 Dr. Harfst wrote a 12-page " Note for Use in the Study of Security Units ". It was circulated to Management Committee members. Once again he revealed a desire and determination " to attain the very highest degree of security that can be mastered ". In two passages he showed a determination to apply an inflexible regime to all patients who entered Cypress,

whether or not in his view they required it as individuals. In two more he showed that he was well aware of the effect of such a policy on some patients.

i. " There is a large group of patients including many persistent sexual offenders who traditionally in the past have been handled (with varying degrees of satisfactoriness) in open wards of hospitals. In South Ockendon Hospital with its 40% level of overcrowding there is no room for them there any more so that any new admissions necessarily have to be to the security unit. It is debatable whether some of them need security in this full sense of the word although they can be handled very well under this regime. I am sometimes questioned by Review Tribunals about the admission of certain types of patient to the unit. I am asked why I cannot relax the secure regime in the ward to allow these patients more individual freedom. I would not admit a case of any sort to Cypress if I did not think at the time that it was appropriate ".

ii. " It is sometimes argued and levelled as a criticism that not all patients in the unit need this level of security and could be allowed to have parole from the ward on a trust basis, the arrangement being withdrawn if the patient abused his privileges. . . There is nothing wrong with a system of trust except that it is in complete contrast to and incompatible with the concept of security. You cannot trust an untrustworthy patient and have security at the same time. The two systems running parallel in the same unit on a long term basis would in my view create irreconcilable precedents and would confuse the staff resulting in overall loss of hard earned gains in security. There comes a time when it is right and proper for certain patients to be given a measure of trust. At this point in time security accommodation becomes inappropriate and I would far sooner transfer the patient to an ordinary hospital ward. *The fact that such vacancies never exist and possibly never will under present circumstances in this hospital is quite immaterial* ". (Our italics).

iii. " If the patients mix freely with those in the rest of the hospital and partake of all the facilities that patients elsewhere in the region enjoy then the unit they live in is only a security unit at night when they return to it. If full security is observed and patients never leave the unit then unless the services of the hospital can be brought to them they suffer accordingly and tend to become an underprivileged group. There are arguments both for and against varying degrees of integration. At South Ockendon Hospital the principle of maximum security attainable has been adhered to which has resulted in patients in the security unit being denied many facilities that the hospital has to offer and has created many further problems in terms of supply of occupational therapy and workshop material, staff distribution and patient living space ". He then goes on to say that he would not favour integration, as the hospital " consists of rather low grade patients in the main " whereas those in Cypress are predominantly high grade. He would rather bring what facilities are available to the unit.

iv. He then deals with the problem of Cypress in relation to " the recidivist offender who possibly after a period of time no longer requires secure accommodation ". He says that this " is a large group and the cause of much difficulty in practice. It is reasonable in most of these cases to recommend after a period of time that they be transferred and rehabilitated (given various positions of graded supervision and trust) on an open ward in the hospital. Unfortunately, no vacancies exist in the rest of the hospital and are likely never to exist in the foreseeable future. . . . They require lifelong supervision in an institutional setting and at the present time the only alternative for them is crippling inactivation due to high security or complete discharge ".

195. At the end of the notes Dr. Harfst clearly posed the problem of the unit's future and suggested a possible alternative use.

196. This paper was not sent to the Board and the only reaction from Management Committee members seems to have been to congratulate him. Dr. Harfst agreed that the occupational facilities on Cypress were extremely limited.

197. On 12 April 1969 the Minister of State visited the hospital with Dr. Brothwood from the Department of Health and Social Security. They held discussions with Dr. Dutton, the Group Secretary and the Chief Male Nurse and later toured the hospital. The Chairman of the Management Committee and Captain Hugh Delargy M.P. were present in the morning. The Department's report of this visit states that it was said of Cypress in the discussions that it was " unsatisfactory because it had no provision for recreation and deprived patients of liberty to a greater degree than a special hospital or prison. . . . There was no element of rehabilitation in their treatment ".

198. In May 1969 the Post Ely Policy Working Party reported on Cypress Villa that " patients cannot be humanely contained, treated, occupied, trained or rehabilitated in a small security unit. They need to have access to training, education, recreation and other facilities ".

199. Before passing on to the arrival of Patient S it is important to try to find some explanation for the unchecked and largely uncommented decline of Cypress from its days under Dr. Dutton to the indignities and rigidity it experienced under Dr. Harfst.

The Effect of Clinical Autonomy

200. Why was nothing said about Dr. Harfst's immediate striking change of policy? Why did nobody seek to modify its worst features?

201· We set out in paragraphs 484–486 the statutory duty of the Secretary of State, the Regional Hospital Board and the Hospital Management Committee. We propose at this stage of our report to look at how some members and officers of the Board and the Management Committee, and some of the consultants and staff saw their position in relation to each other. Where possible we shall look at these attitudes in the context of Cypress Villa, and later we shall see how they affected the position of Patient S and his mother and brother. We do not apologise for setting out the views of a number of the witnesses in some detail, for we were told more than once during the inquiry that the boundaries of clinical autonomy have bedevilled the hospital services for a long time. It seems to us important to recognise the problems that this lack of definition has raised in the past in order that people can see how far the new Management Plans for 1974 have removed them.

The Regional Hospital Board and its officers

202. *Sir Graham Rowlandson* has been Chairman of the Board for 17 years and has been to Cypress Villa on two or three occasions in the course of visits to the South Ockendon Group of Hospitals. One of these visits took place on 16 September 1968. He was accompanied by Mr. Phipps. Sir Graham's written report of this visit set out the purpose of Cypress Villa as being " To provide secure conditions for the treatment of thirty severely disturbed male patients who, while not requiring the maximum security of a Special Hospital, could not be nursed in ordinary hospital conditions ". He then recorded that he had spoken to Dr. Harfst and Dr. Dutton, and that the latter had drawn his attention to the inadequate space for occupational therapy and that they had discussed as possible solutions enclosing the central exercise yard, building an extension to the day rooms and alternative uses for the existing day rooms. This section of Sir Graham's report ended " because of the need to maintain absolute security these suggestions involved problems, particularly regarding the delivery of materials for the type of heavy work—e.g. brick making—most suitable for these patients. It was understood that the Hospital Management Committee would give further consideration to the matter ".

203. Sir Graham was asked about the contrast between the absolute security he found and the medium security which had been the aim.

Q. " At that particular time, were you concerned about Cypress when you saw it ? " A. " It depends exactly what you mean by concerned. It did not seem to me, knowing hospitals, to be a hospital ward. It was a security wing, and rather frightening, with few windows, or windows high up, and therefore visiting hospitals it struck me as very unusual. But this was really a technical problem on which I was not qualified to judge, and I had to accept that the Department and those concerned felt that this was required for this particular kind of patient . . . ".

Q. " Did it appear to you from the answers to your questions that people appeared to know what they were doing ? " A. " I felt so, this is the view I felt. It was comparatively new, we had been requested, as far as I recollect, to do it by the Department. It had been agreed that this was the way to deal with this particular kind of patient, . . . Dr. Harfst, of course was responsible, and he seemed to understand the patients and was dealing with them. I felt at this stage I had to wait and see whether what was felt right turned out to be right . . . ".

Q. " Is it possible for you to deal in any detail with matters that have happened over the many years you have been Chairman of the Board ? " A. " I think this ought to be made clear: I am a lay Chairman of the Board. . . . As I see the Board's function it is to take the policy decisions, and, if I may say so, we are served in my view with really good officers, and my job is really to see that the Board takes proper policy decisions, based, of course, on the views of the Secretary of State for the time being, and then to see they are carried out. I would submit this is what has happened ".

204. Later in his evidence he was questioned further about Cypress.

Q. " I was wondering whether, at the time of your visit in 1968, you had it in mind that orginally the intention was a medium security unit within the Board's area and that what you found was a unit of what is there described [in your Report] as ' absolute security ' ? " A. " I do not think as

54

a lay Chairman I can really express a view on that. My recollection on that was that, apart from wanting us to set up a unit for this type of patient, all I could do as a layman was to try to ascertain that it was being run by someone competent to do so, and then see what the results were ".

Q. " . . . if you saw at a hospital you visited a use for a particular unit which you felt was not the use that the Board provided it for, what course would you then follow ? " A. " I should ask my Senior Administrative Medical Officer to advise me medically and professionally as to what the circumstances were ".

205. Finally he was asked by a member of the Committee " You went to Cypress and you asked questions did you not ? " A. " A lot of questions ".

Q. " Then you said you could not assess whether conditions were suitable in Cypress because this was a medical matter, or words to that effect ? " A. " That is right ".

Q. " . . . did you ask, or were you told, of the precise use of the side rooms, that all patients on admission were put in there possibly for an indefinite period, maybe a day maybe longer and deprived of all reasonable facilities ? Were you told this ? " A. " Yes, this I happen to remember although it is all those years ago . . . I can remember going round a side corridor and actually looking into these various rooms, or I might have been looking through a window. It was alien to our hospital concepts, but having formed those lay views, I did not like the look of the building or the concept of the building, but I understood these were more or less dangerous, psychotic patients, I believe that this is the word. Again, I am a layman, but I had to accept that it was necessary to restrict the liberty of these patients in this way for medical reasons. I did not think I was competent to judge whether it was necessary ".

Q. " But you were not told they were put in there, whether they needed it or not, it was a routine procedure, were you ? " A. " I have almost an impression that it might have been while you assess the patient, but I would not like to be absolutely dogmatic about that ".

206. *Professor Ramsay* was asked at the outset of his evidence about the view he took of his job as Senior Administrative Medical Officer. He regarded himself as adviser to the Board on its hospital specialist services. " I had a special responsibility with respect to the performance of the consultants' work in the sense that I had to report to the Board on this but I was not responsible for the clinical performance of their work by the consultants . . . If the work was not at any time being performed at what one would regard as a reasonable standard I had special responsibility to report to the Board and suggest there was *prima facie* evidence to justify further enquiry by an appropriate committee set up by the Board. Only in those circumstances was I able to intervene in the clinical work of consultants ".

207. Professor Ramsay held the view that there was an important distinction between his role and that of the Board before and after H.M.(69)59 which was sent to all Regional Hospital Boards and Hospital Management Committees in July 1969 following the report on Ely Hospital (Cmnd. 3687). In that memorandum Boards and Committees were reminded that Boards carried out their functions as agents of the Secretary of State and that Management Committees carried out their functions as agents for the Boards, and that, although Manage-

55

ment Committees should exercise their functions without unnecessary intervention by the Boards or Secretary of State, Boards were responsible to the Secretary of State for the service in their areas. The Secretary of State " looks to the Boards to exercise general oversight of the administration and standards of care in the hospital service in their regions, including whatever arrangements for visiting they consider appropriate for this purpose ".

208. Professor Ramsay said that before July 1969 " the Board had an overall responsibility, but did not have day to day monitoring responsibility subsequently imposed on the Board by the then Secretary of State ". He said " monitor means to me that one has to see how the patients are treated. One has to look over a consultant's shoulder. This is a very considerably greater responsibility than was the case prior to 1969 ". When he was asked how he could carry out his pre-1969 responsibility for the performance of consultants' work without just such monitoring, he drew the distinction between taking some action if a complaint reached him and taking the initiative himself to find out whether things were going satisfactorily. Before July 1969 he relied upon complaints. After July 1969 he himself had to take the initiative.

209. Professor Ramsay was asked to define more precisely the word " monitor " which is so freely used at this time. He explained in the context of his responsibility for the performance of consultants' work " It means as I understand it to see that the job is being properly done and to advise the Board, the employing authority, if it is not being properly done . . . I do not believe, even now, the Senior Administrative Medical Officer has any direct responsibility to take steps to ensure the job is being properly done. He would do this through his Board. He is an adviser to his Board, he is not a medical superintendent ".

210. Professor Ramsay then turned to consider the position of the Physician Superintendent. " He is responsible to the Board and to the Management Committee. To the Board he is responsible for his own performance as a consultant psychiatrist. He is the medical administrator who would liaise directly with the Senior Administrative Medical Officer. There must be a dialogue between the two on all matters concerning care of patients in the hospital. As a Physician Superintendent he is the adviser of the Management Committee on services provided by the Management Committee in the hospital ". His responsibility within the hospital for other consultants " is extremely delicate. With good sense and goodwill it is fairly easy to manage and comprehend. The individual clinical care of patients must remain the responsibility of individual consultants. This is a position we cannot depart from. The consultant is responsible to the Board for the individual care of every patient in his charge. The Superintendent has a responsibility for the ambience or environment of the hospital, but not individual care of patients. . . . In a psychiatric hospital the Superintendent should see that the services are in general co-ordinated. This applies to nursing, medical, grounds, gardening, decor. He has an overall responsibility for anything which affects patient welfare but not the individual care of patients ". He was asked where he drew the line between individual care and overall responsibility for the hospital, and was reminded that some witnesses, including Dr. Dutton, had said that everything that went on in the villa, the patients' home, was within the clinical care of the individual consultant. He replied " It is a difficult line to draw. It is not a matter of black and white. It is a matter of shading. Every case which is a borderline case between the Superintendent's responsibility and the

consultant's responsibility must be taken on its merits . . . It is a matter of two colleagues of seniority and standing working together . . . There is no precise guidance over this . . . Every Superintendent has a different relationship with his consultants. The pattern is that which is established as between two colleagues of equal standing and will be different as between any two colleagues ". He agreed that the individuals " formed their own yardstick " and that this yardstick varied from hospital to hospital. He was asked " how does one consultant or one medical man coming from one hospital to another find out, except by bitter experience, that a different yardstick is being applied? " A. " This is how it has operated ever since I have been associated with medical practice. It is even more so in general practice where the doctor is completely autonomous ".

211. Professor Ramsay was then asked when he would expect a Physician Superintendent to report to him matters concerning a consultant in his hospital. He said " There are three circumstances where he should do this on a formal basis. . . . If he has reason to believe that the professional work of one of his colleagues has fallen below a reasonable standard, whatever reasonable means, or if he believes his colleague is unable to carry out his work properly, either because of ill-health or professional incompetence . . . The Senior Medical Officer has to investigate the allegations, but even he has no disciplinary power. His duty is to advise his Board, if there is a *prima facie* case, to set up an appropriate professional committee . . . which would then determine whether there was professional incompetence or not. In the case of ill-health there is a different circular which allows the Senior Administrative Medical Officer to call for an independent medical examination to determine the degree of ill-health of a consultant. . . . On an informal basis without telling tales a consultant can always approach a Senior Medical Officer and express concern and seek advice. The advice is usually almost invariably to stick to the rules laid down. I would never advise consultants to proceed other than in accordance with the rules. It is too dangerous for them, for me, for the service ".

212. The distinction between an acute hospital and South Ockendon was put before Professor Ramsay by a member of the Committee. " On the question of clinical autonomy, it seems readily understandable that in an acute hospital the daily regime of a patient who is there for a comparatively short time should fall fairly and squarely under the single responsibility of a single man. . . . It seems less easy to follow the logic behind handing over every facet of the daily regime of the patient to a single man for what could be a very long period, virtually without challenge. . . . Would you not feel that the two situations are so different that there should be different approaches? " A. " I can see the force of your argument. I am bound to say, though, that as psychiatry develops so the individual responsibility of consultants has to go up with it. . . . Today . . . I do not think any psychiatrist would accept any constraint on how he treats his patients by a Physician Superintendent or a S.A.M.O. He is an independent professional man who should use his independent professional judgment whether dealing with long-stay or short-stay patients ".

213. Professor Ramsay felt that the position was much more sensible since July 1969 although " frankly, most of us do not like the monitoring role . . . The system will never be perfect so long as consultants feel, perhaps rightly, that they must be a little careful what they say about their colleagues ".

214. The same member of the Committee renewed his theme. " If a single consultant has full authority over every facet of a patient's life, is this procedure not too clumsy? " A. " It is a very clumsy procedure. . . . The law of libel comes into this, one has to be so careful. Nevertheless, I believe if one presses these things home, and every S.A.M.O. does press them home, you can arrive, somewhat slowly, at the point of resolution of most problems ".

Q. " But this is not satisfactory, is it, if the patient is confined, perhaps unnecessarily in a side room without care? If you have to go through all this rather clumsy procedure he might be there for weeks on end? " A. " I am afraid so, but may I with respect point out that if a surgeon decides to operate on a patient there is no-one to say that the operation he carries out is necessarily the right one. . . . The patient puts his trust in that surgeon, and he carries out the operation as he thinks best. This is a matter of professional probity ".

215. We now set out how his views affected Professor Ramsay on his visit to Cypress in 1968. It will be recalled that he said that it looked like a prison and did not look the sort of unit he would have wished to be in one of the Board's hospitals. He went on to say that he was not aware that patients were not leaving the villa for occupational therapy. " Nor did I ask the question which I might have done. I would have done if I had been charged with a monitoring role which was imposed on the Board in 1969 ". In answer to the suggestion " Surely one of the purposes of your visit to Cypress in 1968 was to see how the security unit was fulfilling its functions ", he replied " This was not the purpose of my visit. I did not go to Ockendon on this occasion to look at Cypress specifically. It was a pastoral visit ". In connection with the report of Sir Graham Rowlandson's visit he was asked if any suggestion was conveyed to Dr. Harfst that patients should be going out to occupational therapy. He said " I did not at this time regard myself as competent to give such advice ".

216. *Mr. Phipps* has been Secretary of the Board since April 1968. He is Secretary to the meetings of the Chairmen of Regional Hospital Boards for England and Wales, and also to the meetings of Secretaries of the Regional Hospital Boards for England and Wales. He serves on various Departmental working parties. With his long and wide experience we felt that he might be able to assist us with his view on what the procedure should be if a Physician Superintendent and a consultant failed to agree, for example, on the use to be made of side rooms. He said that the Physician Superintendent would then refer the matter informally to the Senior Administrative Medical Officer and that joint discussions would then resolve the dispute. If they failed to do so he did not know what the next step would or should be.

217. Of his visit to Cypress with Sir Graham in September 1968 he said that he was not surprised to find that it had become a unit of absolute security in place of the medium security unit that had been intended. " I regarded this as essentially a medical matter in which I as a layman was not in a position to comment ".

The Hospital Management Committee and its Consultants

218. *Mr. Nichols*, the Chairman of the Hospital Management Committee, said in his written statement that the Management Committee had no juris-

diction in clinical matters except in the case of a complaint made concerning the treatment given to any patient.

219. Mr. Nichols said that he had no idea that security was so tight in Cypress until after the complaints by Patient S's mother towards the end of September 1969. He then asked Dr. Harfst why Patient S was being kept in a side room and was told that it was for assessment purposes. He accepted that that was a matter of clinical judgment. He also regarded the question as to whether there should be a bed or divan or only a mattress on the floor in a side room as being one for clinical judgment, likewise whether a patient should have a cord in his pyjama trousers. Whether a patient should have elastic to hold up his pyjama trousers was not clinical judgment and when the Management Committee knew the position following the complaint by Patient S's mother they recommended that this should be provided. He was asked if he thought that the provision of seats in a side room was a matter for clinical judgment. He said he understood that that provision was also made after the complaint, but he added " I have visited the unit from its inception and I must say the decor was pleasant. It was not a cell, but a side room. It is surely up to the psychiatrist concerned with the welfare of the patients there, or the physician, to give a positive answer when you pose questions as to the reason why these circumstances obtained. I have told you the reason as given, namely, that it was a period of assessment for the safety of the patient ".

220. *Mr. Whiting*, the Vice-Chairman of the Hospital Management Committee, said that he had visited Cypress on " quite a number of occasions when interviewing patients who had applied to the Mental Health Tribunal for discharge from an order. I can only say that in my judgment, as a fairly, I hope, mature person, that nothing I saw then struck me as particularly extreme in the way of regimentation. Dr. Harfst himself was always extremely helpful. I have never known Dr. Harfst socially, but I had quite a lot of talks with him and on all those occasions I felt his attitude towards the patients in Cypress Villa was an extremely sympathetic one ". In a subsequent letter to the Committee Mr. Whiting wrote " Cypress was not wanted by the H.M.C. . . . . We were told that a highly trained expert in forensic psychiatry had been engaged to run it. We had no hand in this appointment made by the R.H.B. Enquiries as to its function and the type of patient brought talk that it was to have relatively high grade psychopaths who needed high security. To me and I think my colleagues this meant people like Neville Heath, Haigh and Straffen for which security would have to be at least as high as Rampton or Moss Side. Personally I do not know how right this is. We accepted that we were in expert Home Office guided hands ".

221. *Dr. Dutton's* letter of appointment as Physician Superintendent said " The duties attached to the post . . . have been broadly defined by the Board as follows:—

Without prejudice to the duties and responsibilities of other members of the Consultant Medical staff of the hospital towards patients under their particular care, the Physician Superintendent shall, in addition to any wards or clinics for which he is personally responsible be broadly responsible for and answerable directly to the Hospital Management Committee for all matters concerning the maintenance of the Medical Services and the overall medical administration of the hospitals. Within the limits of the powers delegated to him, he should have ultimate responsibility for determining the nature, scale, co-ordination and method of functioning of the Therapeutic Services of the hospitals. This would include co-ordination of the nursing services in consultation with the Matrons and the Chief Male Nurse; co-ordination of the work of the medical staff; responsibility for the work of the supplementary medical departments; and establishing liaison with the Local Health Authorities and General Practitioners ".

222. There is no doubt that Dr. Dutton was very glad to hand over Cypress to Dr. Harfst, but in our view he too readily embraced the idea that his successor's one year's experience in a State Hospital in Scotland had given him an expertise which he did not in fact possess. For example, he was writing in November 1967 " We now have a ' forensic psychiatrist ' on the staff who has a lot of experience of security units ". Dr. Dutton acknowledged in evidence that he knew the condition in which patients existed in the side rooms. He said " This was a regime that I accepted. It was a regime provided by a consultant who was experienced and who had worked in a special hospital. It was a regime that I accepted ". He was asked " is there any part of a patient's daily life and routine within a ward which would not in your view come within the clinical care or the clinical judgment of the consultant? " to which he replied " in the field of mental handicap I do not think there is. The total care is the responsibility of the consultant ".

223. Dr. Dutton told us that when he investigated the complaints by Patient S's mother he discovered things that were not acceptable to him, but he did not suggest to Dr. Ramsay or the Hospital Management Committee when they were investigating the mother's complaint that he in any way differed from Dr. Harfst. He said " Dr. Harfst was the consultant who knew the patient. . . . I had no reason to call in doubt Dr. Harfst's judgment ".

224. Dr. Dutton did not agree that he knew that side rooms were being used for punitive purposes before the complaints by Patient S's mother in September 1969. We are satisfied that he must have known of this practice from at least May 1968 when Patient WW was confined to a side room for complaining that a member of the staff had stolen his cigarettes (See paragraphs 563 to 566). We are satisfied that he never remonstrated with Dr. Harfst about this practice. Indeed, we accept Dr. Harfst's evidence that from the discussions he had with Dr. Dutton and others from time to time he thought he was doing the job in a manner which was acceptable to them.

225. Dr. Dutton told us that he himself would at the time of the inquiry run Cypress on rather less rigid lines than it was then being run by Dr. Harfst. He is no longer the Physician Superintendent. He is now the Chairman of the Medical Executive Committee. The following questions and answers followed.

Q. " Has there been any discussion of your view as Chairman of the Medical Executive Committee that it is a little too rigid? " A. " No ".

Q. " In what circumstances would you as Chairman of the Medical Executive Committee be prepared to instigate a discussion at that Committee about a regime under the control of another consultant? " A. " This is very difficult ".

Q. " But it is right at the core, is it not, of keeping acceptable policy in the hospital and acceptable standards? " A. " Yes. One discusses this with one's colleagues because the consultant has his own right to treat patients; he is the one person responsible for the treatment of patients. In the field of mental handicap the regime is part of the therapy. To discuss in committee the way a consultant is running his unit is the same as asking in a general hospital about a discussion between two consultants whether they will give a patient Aldomet or Guanethidine. This is part of the treatment. I am not sure at what level I would in fact discuss this at a Medical Executive Committee meeting. Obviously one discusses this with him on a face to face basis from time to time. I do not think I have discussed this formally with him at all. Frequently the whole ethos of different wards is discussed. This is almost a day to day occurence ".

Q. " It is awfully easy for the reality to disappear submerged beneath words like ' ethos ' and ' face to face ' and ' informal ' and so on. I would just like to understand if I can the kind of circumstances in which you as Chairman of the Medical Executive Committee would raise with the Medical Executive Committee for discussion a regime on a villa which you thought after discussion was too rigid? . . . ". A. " I do not think I would raise it with the Medical Executive Committee ".

He said that he would only raise this with the Board.

226. *Dr. York-Moore* is a consultant at the hospital. At one time he was Physician Superintendent of a hospital in Scotland. He was asked " You have certain problem wards in the hospital, one of which is Cypress, which we gather is (now) a dumping ground for the rest of the hospital. How much of a common approach is there between the consultants to try and work through this problem? Or do you see it as being something that Dr. Harfst, as the consultant responsible for that ward, is lumbered with and left to paddle his own canoe? " A. " I think inevitably in medical work—and you are not going to like this because I am going to use terms you do not like—there are areas of clinical responsibility, and one of the ways in which we hold each other in respect is by respecting precisely those . . . ".

Q. " You have said why you think, from a medical point of view, that it is a good thing. But can you help me from my layman point of view? What you say you think is a good thing would seem to me personally . . . a system that might perhaps withhold support and encouragement when support and encouragement may be most needed? " A. " You may be right. I do not think it is an easy situation to sum up in a sentence ".

227. He went on to explain that you can only give help when you feel that you have something to offer. " It is not much good saying to someone who has got a problem ' Bad luck, old chap, I wish I could help ', and in fact offering nothing ".

Q. " That is really why I pressed my questions on this, saying so far as a problem ward like Cypress is concerned, is there a common approach and discussion among consultants together of the problems of that particular ward? " A. " No, there has not been. As far as I can remember, there was not a staff meeting as such. We tended to talk more about the general problems that we were confronted with rather than the specific one at such meetings, because the question of overcrowding was not restricted to Cypress particularly ".

228. He agreed that the medical profession place great reliance on the integrity of individual consultants and are chary of doing or saying anything which might appear to be casting doubt upon a consultant's ability.

229. *Dr. Harfst* was also questioned about his view of the responsibility of the consultant. He agreed that when he applied for the job of consultant at South Ockendon Hospital the job specification included: " There will shortly be opened a new unit for the treatment of male subnormal psychopaths under conditions of security. This is to be run on therapeutic lines and the consultant appointed will be expected to participate actively in the dynamic approach to the treatment of this class of patient ".

Q. " You as the consultant would be the person responsible for setting up the regime within these general limits? " A. " Yes ".

Q. " It was your job to provide yourself with the guidelines? " A. " Yes ".

Q. " The position of the consultant is one in which you would expect to be able to take decisions, and quite fundamental decisions, in relation to the running of this unit, on your own? " A. " Yes ".

230. Later in the evidence he was asked

Q. " When you were confronted by the ward, and having seen it as run by Dr. Dutton, did you get in touch with the Board or the Board's officers themselves to raise any queries with them about the ward and what was to be done with it? " A. " No ".

Q. " Would it be right to say that you felt rightly or wrongly that your job as the consultant was to do what you felt was right with what you had been given? " A. " Yes, I did. I felt the pressure was on me to do something, not to complain ".

231. Somewhat later he was questioned about accepting responsibility for the patients in his care.

Q. " And matters of clinical policy are, in general terms, your responsibility in relation to those patients? " A. " Yes ".

Q. " But within the hospital set up there is the Medical Executive Committee? " A. " Yes ".

Q. " And on that Committee the consultants and the medical staff discuss general medical and clinical matters, is that right? " A. " They do not discuss clinical matters ".

Conclusions as to why the regime in Cypress was permitted to develop in the manner described earlier

232. In our view the most important factor was the reluctance of all concerned to say or do anything which might be thought to be calling a consultant's decision into question. It was an attitude of mind which prevented a true mutli-disciplinary approach to the hospital's planning and problems at all levels. It operated on the minds of people in varying ways.

i. Sir Graham Rowlandson did not like the restriction of liberty that he found, but felt that he had to accept the medical justification put forward. " I am only a layman ".

ii. Mr. Nichols too readily succumbed to the explanation that the un-dignified, unjustifiable side room regime was necessary for the assessment and safety of new patients. We consider that the mystique of the consultant was so potent that obvious questions were not asked because the way of life in the villas was regarded as being entirely within the consultant's control. Any examination of the ward report books would have revealed the use of the side rooms for punishment, but we do not think it occurred to the Management Committee members to look at them for the same reason. Any misgivings Mr. Whiting had were calmed by the belief that the patients were men like Neville Heath, Haigh and Straffen.

iii. Dr. Ramsay would have found out in 1968 that patients were not going out for occupational therapy or making use of any other hospital facilities if he had asked about this during his visit to Cypress. But he asked no questions on this topic because, in our view, he too attached overdue importance to the clinical autonomy of the consultant.

iv. Dr. Dutton permitted a complete reversal of his own policy to occur without, so far as we could discover, a word of disapproval to anyone. Again the explanation was the clinical autonomy of the consultant.

v. Dr. York-Moore's attitude to clinical responsibility in our view was a barrier to the initiation of discussions between consultants which would have given Dr. Harfst the support and advice which he needed, but which it was not his nature to seek.

vi. Dr. Harfst considered himself responsible for setting up the regime in Cypress and for taking decisions on his own.

233. Because of this insistence upon the supremacy of the consultant responsible for the villa there were no multi-disciplinary meetings, as there should have been, to discuss the kind of patient to be admitted, the kind of care and treatment that should and could be provided, the manner in which the villa would be run, how the problems foreseen by Dr. Dutton would be overcome and the equipment required. Dr. Dutton should have convened one such meeting before the villa opened and another when Dr. Harfst joined the hospital. They should have been attended by all the consultants, the medical staff attached to the villa, the Head of Nursing Services, the Group Secretary, the Hospital Secretary, the Head of Occupational Therapy and the Head of Industrial Therapy. A clear policy directive should have been worked out and written down. If these meetings had been held the mistakes that followed would probably have been avoided. We consider in Chapter X of this report a formal multi-disciplinary structure for the hospital and how a true multi-disciplinary approach affects a consultant's position in a subnormality hospital.

234. The Management Committee members should have insisted on much more information than they were given. Without a clearer understanding of what kind of patients were going to be admitted and how it was going to be run the Management Committee could not know whether it had sufficient equipment. The officers of the Group and the Chairman of the Management Committee had a joint responsibility to see that it was given sufficient information.

235. Lay people at all levels of the administration and management failed to put sufficient trust in their instinct that something was wrong. They appear to have distrusted the evidence of their own eyes. If a member of a Committee or an administrator feels that something is wrong in a hospital he must ask questions until he is satisfied. We found a regrettable tendency either to ask no questions or to accept the first answer that was given " because this is a medical matter and I am only a layman ". This would not have mattered if Dr. Ramsay or Dr. Dutton had shown any greater willingness to ask the questions that they should undoubtedly have been asking.

Patient S

236. S was born on 12 September 1929. He was admitted to Stoke Park Hospital, Bristol, as a subnormal patient in 1939. He was licensed to the care of his mother in September 1951, but was readmitted to the hospital in January 1952. In 1956 he was transferred to the Royal Earlswood Hospital at Redhill. He was released to the care of his mother shortly after and held various jobs in the catering trade. He is of frail physique and has very poor eyesight. During the years 1961 to 1968 he had five convictions for indecent assaults on children and was dealt with by way of conditional discharge, probation, and committals to hospital. Following his conviction in 1968 he was admitted to Darenth Park Hospital in Kent under Section 60 of the Mental Health Act 1959. After a year as an inpatient he was released on trial leave to his mother on 25 July 1969.

237. On 8 August S indecently assaulted an eight year old girl by tickling her on her waist and on the outsides of her thighs. When she began to cry he stopped. He was admitted to Wandsworth Prison to await trial before the Recorder of Southend-on-Sea on 16 September 1969. On 22 August the Medical Officer of the prison telephoned South Ockendon Hospital to enquire whether they had a place for S who, in his opinion, was in need of hospital treatment. He was told that the hospital was admitting no new patients. The Medical Officer subsequently got in touch with Dr. Harfst and put strong pressure on him to admit S saying that the alternative would be a prison sentence. Dr. Harfst therefore went to interview him at the prison and studied his case records. Unfortunately, Dr. Harfst somehow got the impression that he had at some time served a two year prison sentence. This was incorrect. Dr. Harfst claimed that there was an entry showing such a sentence in the records at Wandsworth Prison. We sent for the records and found that his recollection was at fault. He agreed to accept S under Section 60 of the Mental Health Act 1959 if the Recorder so ordered. Both he and the Prison Medical Officer submitted reports to the Court in which they said S was suffering from subnormality which warranted his detention in a hospital for medical treatment. That from the latter stated " He needs to be cared for in a stable and secure environment ". That from Dr. Harfst said " In my opinion he requires a further period of compulsory supervision in a subnormality hospital and I would recommend that a restriction be placed on his discharge from a compulsory order without limit of time ".

238. Dr. Harfst attended the Court on 16 September and gave evidence in accordance with his report. He left before sentence was passed. He did not tell the Recorder that the vacancy reserved for S had to be in the security unit. Neither did he take the opportunity of speaking to the mother and brother of S. In passing sentence the Recorder, Mr. Malcolm Morris Q.C., said that his duty

to the public and his desire to assist S did not conflict, and he made an order under Section 60 of the Mental Health Act 1959 admitting him to South Ockendon Hospital for treatment and imposed an order under Section 65 restricting his discharge for an unlimited period. He went on: " that, I would like to make absolutely clear, does not involve your staying in that hospital one moment longer than the doctors think is necessary but gives them the absolute discretion, should you not do as well as they hope. I hope you will. You are somebody who is obviously longing to live an ordinary life at home and staying with your mother and brother, and I hope it will not be too long before you are doing so, but you must appreciate, as I am sure they do, that for the moment what you need is help from the doctors, and I wish you luck ". The Recorder formed a favourable view of S's mother and took the very unusual step of committing him to her care, instead of to the police, to deliver to the hospital.

239. S had never absconded from any hospital and there was nothing in any previous reports to suggest that he might have suicidal or violent or homosexual tendencies. We are satisfied that it was unnecessary for S to be admitted to any security unit, let alone one with the characteristics of Cypress at that time.

240. Dr. Harfst told us that he had no particular care or form of treatment in mind. " I thought eventually simple ordinary hospital care for a period. I hoped not for too long ". He was then asked if he thought at that time that he could offer him suitable treatment for rehabilitation in Cypress, and replied " I felt I could not offer him the entire treatment for rehabilitation he needed in Cypress, but I felt, in view of the fact that I thought his hospital admission was necessary, it was reasonable that he should go to Cypress Villa in the first instance ". He said that he thought it might be necessary for S to remain in Cypress for three to six weeks at the end of which he felt sure that he would be suitable for an open ward.

241. We are satisfied that Dr. Harfst's recollection is at fault. It is clear from his paper of February 1969 that he can never have had any real prospect of transferring S to another ward.

242. We propose to set out in chronological order the events that followed as we find them to have occurred.

16 September

243. In the afternoon S was taken by his mother and brother to the hospital. After some delay Dr. Harfst arrived at the Administration office and directed them to take S to Cypress Villa. The mother asked " Do you want to know anything about S? " and Dr. Harfst said " No ". The brother said of that conversation " The thing that struck me most was the unco-operativeness of Dr. Harfst. He just did not want to know anything. He literally shrugged his shoulders ". We accept that he gave this impression to the relatives.

244. When they reached the villa they were well received by the charge nurse and given a cup of tea. The mother and brother were told that S could wear his own clothing, that he could smoke if he wished to, that he could keep his personal belongings and that he would be allowed to work. Although the mother was apprehensive about the constant locking of doors the brother tried to reassure her after they had left. Dr. Benton, who was the Duty Medical Officer, carried

out a brief examination of S and had some conversation with the mother. It is clear from her note that the mother was concerned about how long S would be " confined " in Cypress and what she could do about it. Dr. Benton tried without success to contact Dr. Harfst. S complained of a headache. The ward reports record that for the remainder of that day and night he was quiet and co-operative. He was confined in the side room in conditions we have already described.

17 September

245. S complained to the staff that his breakfast wasn't very good and that he would tell his brother who would make it difficult for the hospital as he worked for the *News of the World*.

19 September

246. S's mother and a friend visited Cypress. They took S's watch, some clothing and some sweets and biscuits. The bell was answered after some minutes and they were at first refused admission as they had come on a weekday without making any arrangement. But the mother who is a determined lady put her foot in the door and managed to get admission. S was brought to her from what she fairly described as a cell. He was wearing a pair of pyjamas without any cord and was without his glasses, slippers or a dressing gown. He was trembling and crying and appeared frightened and cold. She asked the nursing staff why he was kept in the cell and was told that he was put there " as any other patient was, to teach them what would happen if they did not behave ". She asked if S had done anything wrong and was told " that will teach him if he does ". It was explained that he had no reading matter " because that was the rule . . . : they took everything away ". The nursing staff would not let her see the side room, but she managed to look in from outside and saw " one small, bare cell with a mattress on the floor, and nothing else ".

247. After leaving the villa she went to the Hospital Secretary. His report described her as somewhat disturbed and overwrought. She burst out " Won't anyone help me? Can't you do something? " He got in touch with Dr. Dutton, who referred her to Dr. Harfst. She described the condition in which she had found S and asked for an explanation. Dr. Harfst said that he was in the side room because he was in an emotional state. She pointed out that he had not yet seen S and he admitted that this was so, but said he knew what was going on. The mother was undoubtedly a very angry and abusive woman as a result of what she had seen and been told. Her anger was entirely justified, her abuse entirely understandable. She described Dr. Harfst as sitting back with his hands in his trouser pockets with an air of derision on his face. She said that his attitude was one of " sheer disinterest ". We accept that he gave this impression. Dr. Harfst's note of the interview a day or two afterwards is revealing. He wrote " My impression was that she was only interested in attacking me and not in making genuine complaints. I told her that I could do nothing to help her in her present state of mind and advised her to take her complaints elsewhere ". He told her that she could not resume her visit to S and issued instructions that she was not to be admitted to the villa again that day.

248. Dr. Harfst said to us that at the time of the interview on 19 September he imagined that S was out of the side room by day and sleeping in it at night.

He had no means of checking on the validity of the mother's complaints without asking the staff about them. He failed to do this and only saw S for the first time three days later on 22 September.

249. S's mother then returned to the Hospital Secretary who spent two hours with her trying to record her complaints. In his written report made seven days later he commented " One could easily dismiss all this as the ramblings of a mentally disturbed person but . . . the facts are basically true, even though they tend to become quite out of proportion when taken out of context and without due regard for the reasons for them. . . . We are well aware of the difficulties of Cypress Ward and, perhaps, would have to agree with [her] that ' it is worse than prison ' in some respects ".

21 September

250. In the afternoon S's brother visited him. The position was much the same as on the 19th. S was still without his glasses. The staff found the brother perfectly polite until the end of the interview when he asked a number of questions about the conditions in which S was being kept, including why had he no socks and why couldn't he smoke or have any sweets. To each question the staff said that they could not answer and referred him to Dr. Harfst. The brother became exceedingly angry. All staff had been instructed by Mr. Laide, the Senior Assistant Chief Male Nurse, to answer all questions from S's relations in this way.

251. Dr. Harfst told us that the staff should have been able to answer such questions as why a patient could not smoke or have any sweets, as those were matters of routine which he left to the nurses' discretion. When he was referred to a report by Mr. Willingham on his file dated 29 September 1969 recording that none of those questions by the brother had been answered Dr. Harfst was unable to account for his failure to take any steps about this departure from normal practice.

22 September

252. The ward report shows that S was seen for the first time by Dr. Harfst on this day. Dr. Harfst could not explain why he had not seen him earlier. The report states " Patient's attitude remains critical towards the staff and also ward regulations generally. Patient to remain in bed until further notice for observation. Allowed up in dressing gown this p.m. for one hour for exercise ". The clinical notes contain a note by Dr. Leek, the Registrar, stating that S was seen by Dr. Harfst, that he complained of " various matters " and was " negative and passively aggressive " and that he was to remain in the side room a little longer. Dr. Harfst told us that he ordered S to remain longer in the side room because he was disturbed. He agreed that this did not accord with the notes made in the Day Report or by Dr. Leek in the clinical notes, and that S only became disturbed at the prospect of another argument between his mother and the staff. We are satisfied that Dr. Harfst ordered S to remain in the side room in order to try to stifle criticism by his mother, brother and himself. He was being used as a pawn in the battle that had developed between Dr. Harfst and the staff, on the one hand, and his relatives, on the other, over the conditions in which he was being kept.

253. On this day S's mother telephoned the Department of Health and Social Security detailing her complaints. These were set out in a letter from the Depart-

ment to the Secretary of the Regional Hospital Board. On 25 September Dr. Ramsay sent a copy of the letter to Dr. Dutton asking for an urgent report.

24 September

254. The ward report states that S was " very subdued this morning: worried what mother will say or do when she next visits. Up for short period this afternoon: seemed brighter, not complaining ".

25 September

255. S's mother visited her son in Cypress and demanded to see a doctor. Dr. Benton, the Duty Medical Officer, was summoned to the villa and interviewed her. Part of Dr. Benton's entry in the clinical notes reads " She requested [the] interview in S's room as she wanted to ask me something about his condition . . . so I complied . . . She demanded [to know] why S was shaking and accused the staff and regime of reducing him to this situation . . . I said there were several possible explanations and no-one could answer immediately. I thought she was creating a state of anxiety in the room—and she promptly repudiated. She demanded to know whether I agreed with the treatment he was receiving, that he had to stay in bed etc. and not have cigarettes and a locker . . . I explained that I was not the responsible Medical Officer but only the duty doctor and that it was not my place to discuss his treatment but I would record her complaints. . . . In my opinion this unfortunate woman is extremely disturbed and it would be quite useless to argue with her. Her manner was domineering, aggressive and offensive. Dr. Harfst was not in the hospital and Dr. Leek was off duty but was contacted by phone and said he did not think any further intervention would help ".

256. Dr. Benton was asked if she thought that it was helpful to deal with the mother's questions by refusing to discuss the matters she was raising. She replied " I think it is very difficult. One cannot discuss it out of relation to the circumstances. It was part of a treatment programme in which I was not intimately concerned at that moment, and I do not think it would have been helpful if one had expressed personal opinions to her when I did not know the full circumstances. I think it would have been unhelpful because it would have been confusing to her. I had every sympathy with her . . . I think one has to accept that sometimes one cannot be helpful at that juncture except by trying to tell her about where to go to find the answers which I was not able to give her ".

257. Dr. Benton said that she was not aware at the time of her interview that S had been kept in a side room for the nine days since his admission although this was one of the mother's complaints. She had only to look in the ward report book to see if this was so. She said that at the time of giving evidence she believed that there were good reasons for keeping S in the side room for this period of time. When she was asked to give those reasons they did not emerge clearly, but we understood her to be saying that they were the difficulties created for the staff by the determination of S's mother and brother to get him out of the villa. When she was asked why it was necessary for patient S to wear pyjamas while he was in the side room she said " I understand that this was part of the security system at that time and . . . however much one might like to make individual

variations I do not think this works, in the sense that one has to keep the whole place, one has to look after other people as well. I think one has to accept these things ".

258. Right at the end of her evidence she was asked whether she thought the mother had some cause to be upset. She replied " Looking at it just on face value, in the face of the circumstances, naturally I do not think anyone likes to see a patient in such conditions ".

Q. " But you would have thought she had some reason to be upset? " A. " I think any mother would be upset ".

Q. " I am not talking about any mother, but this particular mother about the conditions her son was in? " A. " No more than anybody would have been in the circumstances ".

Q. " But you did not feel it necessary to go and talk over the case perhaps with Dr. Harfst or other medical opinion because you did not think there was enough in her complaint to warrant it? Would that be right? " A. " No, because I thought her complaint had to be seen in relation to the total situation ".

Q. " The total situation, so far as I can see, was that this man had just been received into hospital, had all his clothes removed, he was kept in a side room without very much in the way of amenities. Why did the total situation demand this? " A. " Because, as I understand it, this was what was felt to be necessary at that time in running Cypress as a security ward ".

26 and 27 September

259. The ward report book recorded that on the 26th S was not complaining and seemed to be settling down, and that on the 27th he was allowed out for one hour's exercise after which he became very nervous. When he was asked why, he said that he thought he was going to have a visit and was worried about what his mother would do.

260. On the 26th Mrs. Protheroe, the Chairman of the Patients and Welfare Sub-Committee, was notified that S's mother had made a complaint to the Department of Health and Social Security.

28 September

261. S's mother and brother visited Cypress. When they asked Mr. Laide about S being confined in a side room and whether they could see where he slept they were told that those questions were for medical decision. They saw a tin of sweets they had previously brought for S on the office table and were told that they were being held for him there.

29 September

262. S's mother and brother had an appointment to see Dr. Dutton at 11.30 a.m. They arrived half-an-hour early and asked if they could see S. The request was conveyed to Dr. Harfst who refused permission. The first part of the interview was conducted by Dr. Dutton alone. It was quiet and polite. Dr. Dutton made a note later that day " [S's mother] was concerned, for in her opinion her son had deteriorated since his admission and she could get no satisfactory explanation as to the need for [him] to be in a locked ward and she felt that her son was being kept in a side room for punishment. [She] reiterated her complaints

about ventilation, lack of slippers, no pyjama girdle, cold food and dirty crockery and calling of her son at night for toilet purposes. They added further complaints about S's glasses being removed from him; no books being provided; the side room lacked a bedstead and there was no furniture in the room. [S's mother] said her son S was afraid that her visits would produce repercussions and his period in the side room would be prolonged ". Dr. Dutton, although sympathetic, said he didn't really know much about it and suggested that Dr. Harfst, the responsible consultant, should come and answer their questions. When he joined them his answers were not acceptable to S's mother and brother. He gave them the impression of leaning back in his chair and sneering, and they became increasingly abusive. When they asked if they could see S before going home Dr. Harfst refused permission. The interview ended by Dr. Dutton saying that he would refer the matter to the Regional Hospital Board officers who would be attending a meeting at the hospital that afternoon.

263. S's mother and brother entered the staff dining room and demanded to see a Regional Hospital Board officer. Dr. Camm, a Principal Assistant Senior Medical Officer with the Board, then spoke to them for about half-an-hour in Dr. Dutton's office. They found him sympathetic and he calmed the situation. He asked Dr. Harfst if they could see S. Initially Dr. Harfst refused but eventually Dr. Camm persuaded him to give permission. Dr. Camm accompanied S's mother and brother to Cypress Villa. In the words of his report written the following day " I found the unshaven, frail 40-year-old man standing on his pallet bed in an unheated side room. His glasses had been returned to him but he had nothing to read. His soft slippers were kept outside his locked room ". Dr. Camm was unable to get any satisfactory explanation from anyone as to why S had been detained in the side room for 14 days, and Dr. Dutton confirmed to him that S's mother had received no satisfactory explanation.

30 September

264. Dr. Dutton wrote to Dr. Ramsay who had asked him for an urgent report. He wrote " The treatment of the patient is the sole responsibility of the consultant in charge of the patient and the Physician Superintendent has no locus in this. The nursing care of the patient in a ward is determined by the consultant in charge who also would determine visiting arrangements ". He recommended that an independent enquiry should consider the matter.

265. Dr. Dutton suggested that the Patients and Welfare Sub-Committee should go to Cypress and assess the position, but its Chairman thought that they should not do this without the approval of the Chairman of the Hospital Management Committee as S's mother had made a complaint to the Department. Unfortunately he was away.

266. S ceased to be confined to the side room by day. Dr. Harfst said that he did not think that this decision was connected with Dr. Camm's visit the day before. We are, however, satisfied that if Dr. Camm had not intervened S would have spent further days in the side room.

1 October

267. Dr. Harfst wrote a long report to Dr. Ramsay seeking to explain away or justify the matters complained of by S's mother. Of the side room regime for new patients he said " All patients on admission to the unit are put to bed in a

single room. This period of management may last several days to several weeks, depending on the mental state of the patient. Efforts are made by the staff during this period to introduce the patient gradually and progressively to the rest of the unit and the other patients in it by giving him increasing periods of time in the main ward during the day. The reason for this regime is twofold: to give the patient a chance to accommodate to his new surroundings in a satisfactory manner, and to give the staff a chance to assess the patient's mental state and potentialities. I do not think such a regime could be described as inhumane. It is calculated to serve the patient's best interests in every way and it is widely practised in special hospitals and, indeed, in some modified form in other hospitals ".

2 October

268. The Group Secretary wrote to S's mother saying that the Hospital Management Committee would like to discuss matters with her and asking her to suggest a convenient place and time.

6 October

269. A special ad hoc committee of the Hospital Management Committee inspected Cypress Villa and received reports from Dr. Harfst and Dr. Dutton. Dr. Harfst, in his letter of 1 October, presented the side room regime as a friendly and essential " running in " period for new patients. In answer to Mrs. Protheroe he said there could be no exception to the rule that he, as the Responsible Medical Officer in charge of the unit, had laid down. It was essential to use a side room to form a preliminary assessment of individual patients with regard to " suicidal propensities, homicidal propensities, violent propensities, homosexuality ". Dr. Dutton told the ad hoc committee that in answer to the mother's complaints on 29 September he " had drawn [her] attention to the fact that Dr. Harfst was the Responsible Medical Officer in this case and therefore had full clinical responsibility for the patients under his care ". At no time did he suggest that he had any misgivings about the regime in Cypress.

8 October

270. S's mother had a long meeting with the ad hoc committee. She spoke to the committee telling them of her complaints and fears for one hour and ten minutes at the outset, and members of the committee then attempted to justify the regime to her, assuring her that there was no element of punishment. Mr. Whiting, the Chairman of the ad hoc committee, told her that the committee were going to consider the provision of fixed divans and seats in the side rooms and either nightshirts or pyjamas with elastic waist bands. He wrote his own report to supplement the official minutes. He concluded " We were, I feel, very patient indeed and forbearing that nobody tried on any occasion to score any points over [her]. She herself agreed that she had on occasions been very distraught and that she had been very rude. I am of the opinion that nothing by way of explanation or any form of appeasement which could be offered to [her] will make any effect upon her. She will be a continual source of grave anxiety both to the medical staff and undoubtedly cause undeserved distress and provocation to the nursing staff. I would strongly recommend that if it is possible for him to be transferred elsewhere, this should be effected at the earliest possible time ".

71

271. It is not surprising that S's mother found this meeting unsatisfactory. She said that she was listened to politely, but that she did not feel that she was believed. The Management Committee members' state of mind was that the regime was justifiable, whereas we agree with S's mother that it was wholly unjustifiable. The Committee members could not accept what S's mother asserted, and we have found to be fact, namely that side rooms were being used to punish patients. The Committee members regarded her admitted outbursts and rudeness as causing unnecessary anxiety, distress and provocation to medical and nursing staff, whereas we regard such conduct as the understandable outbursts of a mother whose questions and complaints had not been answered or acted upon.

272. On this day the Recorder of Southend-on-Sea wrote to the Secretary of the Regional Hospital Board sending all the documents dealing with the offence for which he had sentenced S, together with a signed statement from S's mother. His letter concluded with these words " If [her] statement is true—and I have no reason to believe it is not—it discloses an appalling state of affairs which calls not only for immediate action in the case of [S] but for a searching inquiry and urgent action to ensure that other patients are not being similarly and quite unnecessarily subjected to what, as a layman in medical matters, I can only regard as utterly inhuman treatment. I have no hesitation in agreeing with Mrs. S that it is not what the Court had in mind when passing sentence ".

9 October
273. Dr. Shapiro, the Medical Superintendent of Harperbury Hospital, visited Cypress at the request of the Regional Hospital Board. He thought the regime was extremely security minded and too rigid. Although he would have admitted S to a locked ward he would not have subjected him to the side room regime. He left feeling that the Board should look into conditions in Cypress Villa. Most unfortunately he did not say this in his letter of 13 October to Dr. Camm. The only comment in that letter which could be construed as criticism was " It did appear to me that the routine of the security ward was somewhat rigid and very security minded. I was informed by Dr. Harfst that this routine was made necessary by the violent and impulsive patients who are normally in the ward, and the lack of staff to man the ward ".

274. On 13 November Dr. Shapiro called on Dr. Camm. He accepted the accuracy of the note made by Dr. Camm on that day. " Dr. Shapiro called at his request to say that he had been very disturbed by conditions in Cypress Ward, South Ockendon Hospital. He felt the regime there to be rigid. He had not, he said, put this opinion in writing because he had not wished any quotation from his letter to attract adverse publicity to South Ockendon Hospital. If, however, he were to be asked in Court if he would himself have treated S as he had been treated at South Ockendon Hospital he would have to say ' no '. Dr. Shapiro hoped the Board would not mind his suggesting that conditions in Cypress Ward should perhaps be investigated ".

12 October
275. S's mother again visited Cypress Villa. An argument ensued with the staff. It is clear from the terms of the charge nurse's note made three days later that he had done nothing to lower the temperature. He wrote " About 3.45 p.m. she demanded a glass of water. I told her ' You can at least say please '. She

refused. I took particular pains to make sure the glass was clean and I gave her the glass of water on a saucer. She did not bother to say thanks . . . As [she] and the patient's brother were about to leave the ward I said to her ' Mrs. S, you asked for a glass of water and you never drank it '. She replied ' Thanks for your water, it was very nice in a dirty glass '. I said, ' In future don't ask me for anything . . . '. In my opinion [her] main purpose in visiting her son is to provoke and demoralise the staff. She is very critical, very demanding, insultive and abusive. I feel it is unfair for the staff and ward in general to have to put up with such behaviour especially in front of other visitors who might think the staff to blame ".

15 October

276. There was a meeting of the ad hoc committee to discuss the complaints by S's mother. The committee was told of the contents of Dr. Shapiro's letter of 13 October, a copy of which had been received from Dr. Camm that morning. It also considered the charge nurse's report of the incidents on 12 October and a request by Dr. Harfst that S's mother should be informed in writing that, unless she modified her behaviour towards the staff, she would not be permitted to visit the hospital. It was agreed that such a letter should be sent and that enquiries should be made into the possibility of installing fixed divans and seats in the side rooms and providing pyjama trousers with elastic tops or nightshirts. It was also agreed " that the most normal procedure had been followed on and after the admission of the patient ".

277. No voice was raised in protest against the suggestion that the letter should be sent to S's mother. Dr. Dutton did not voice any of the doubts which he told us that he had about the regime. Dr. Harfst sent a short, sharply expressed letter to S's mother on the following day.

16 October

278. A note of a telephone message received from S's mother was passed to Dr. Harfst. She wished to know if she could take S out of the hospital for treatment from his own dentist, and asked if the hospital would telephone her with the answer so that she could make arrangements. Dr. Harfst wrote at the bottom that he had no power to allow parole outside the hospital grounds " The answer is *no*. I see *no reason* why we should telephone [S's mother] for any but purposes suitable for us ".

279. Dr. Harfst told us that it was written under stress and was regrettable.

22 October

280. Dr. Harfst's uncompromising and abrasive attitude towards S's mother is again conveyed very clearly by a note he prepared of an encounter with her on this day.

281. " She stopped me in the corridor of the Administration Block after her visit. She had no appointment. She asked me if she could donate a bed to the hospital so that her son could use it in the side room on Cypress. I replied that no exception could be made for her son. She asked how long he would continue to sleep on the floor. I replied that he would probably be moved to the dormitory very soon but he seemed upset at the moment ' by a family bereavement '. She

said ' he was upset simply because he had to sleep on the floor and this upset her as well '. She said she preferred to call the side room private rooms and asked if her son could not be allowed to stay there rather than the dormitory provided he had a proper bed to sleep on. I said he could not. She said ' Can you spare me a few minutes or am I taking up your time ? ' I replied that she was doing the latter. She then said ' Oh, thank you very much ' and walked off quickly to her car. Her behaviour was more controlled on this occasion than hitherto, her general manner instead displaying gross impudence ".

282. When Dr. Harfst was asked before us to explain why the offer of the bed could not be accepted he replied " I felt that the offer was one made really to embarrass me, not for any other real reason ". He went on to say that he could not see any special reason why an exception should be made and ward routine departed from.

29 October
283. Dr. Harfst discovered that S's mother had left him a cup which he kept in his locker and used in preference to ward crockery. He instructed the staff not to permit S to use the cup and to ask his mother to remove it. He explained to us " The staff themselves were very keen not to use it. They felt that this was another challenge from [S's mother] and they asked me to give authority not to use it and I gave it to support them ". He told us that if a relation had brought a cup for use by any other patient he would have raised no objection.

284. On the same day S's mother while visiting Cypress asked the charge nurse for some cups as she had forgotten to bring some with her thermos of tea. The charge nurse refused to let her have the cups and reminded her that she had not drunk the water he had provided on a previous occasion.

30 October
285. S's mother wrote and asked Dr. Harfst what treatment S was receiving. He replied on 2 December that it was nursing care and supervision. He told us that he had considered psychological treatment but rejected it as he did not think that the patient had sufficient motivation or ability to co-operate. He also considered drug treatment and held it in reserve. There is no reference to any consideration of such treatment in the patient's file.

16 November
286. Dr. Ramsay submitted a long written report to the Finance and General Purposes Committee of the Regional Hospital Board. He concluded " In summary it would seem that S's mother's chief allegations relate to facts and in the main are not disputed. Their interpretation is, however, open to doubt since the conditions of which she complained are associated with the patient's clinical condition and treatment which is largely the responsibility of the Consultant in charge of the case ". He recommended that discussions be held with the Department and the Hospital Management Committee on whether it was necessary to continue to use Cypress as a Regional Security Unit.

21 November
287. The Secretary of the Regional Hospital Board wrote a long letter to S's mother. He concluded by saying that the Board accepted her chief complaints.

" They (the Board) are satisfied, however, that these conditions are associated with the patient's clinical condition and treatment, and they note that the Consultant in charge was not aware of the Court's intention in the matter. They are pleased that the clinical view is now that S is suitable for transfer to an open ward and would like to assure you that arrangements for this are being most urgently pursued. As soon as a vacancy is offered in a hospital outside the Region, the Home Office's consent will be sought for his transfer. The Board, the Senior Administrative Medical Officer and I greatly regret that you have been distressed by circumstances attending S's detention in hospital on a Court Order and we hope that you will feel reassured following this very full enquiry ".

29 November

288. S was transferred to Oaks Villa.

Early December

289. The Regional Hospital Board decided that Cypress should no longer be used as a security unit for the region.

12 January 1970

290. S was transferred to Cell Barnes Hospital.

Conclusions

291.   i. Every aspect of S's existence in the side room was totally unjustifiable. We agree with the Recorder's comment that it was " utterly inhuman treatment ".

  ii. The anger of his mother when she observed those conditions was inevitable and just. The refusal of the nursing staff and of Dr. Benton to answer even simple questions understandably led her to become abusive.

  iii. The failure of Dr. Harfst to see S until 22 September is inexcusable, particularly in view of the complaints by the mother to him on 19 September.

  iv. Dr. Harfst's instructions on 22 September that S should remain longer in the side room were unjustified and inexcusable. In part he was using S as a weapon in his battle with the mother who had right on her side, and in part he was seeking to stifle S's legitimate criticism of the conditions in which he was being held.

  v. S would not have been let out of the side room by day on 30 September if it had not been for Dr. Camm's intervention.

  vi. Dr. Dutton failed to do or say anything useful. Although he had heard from Dr. Ramsay of S's mother's complaint to the Department at least three days before 29 September he was quite unable to give Dr. Camm any explanation for the conditions in which S was being held. Whatever he felt to be the limitations on his powers of corrective action he should have made fuller enquiries than he did.

  vii. If Dr. Dutton was unhappy, as he claimed, about certain aspects of the regime in Cypress it was, in our opinion, his duty as Physician Superintendent to let both the ad hoc committee and Dr. Ramsay know his views. He told neither.

viii. If Dr. Shapiro had put in his letter of 13 October what he subsequently told Dr. Camm a month later, it is unlikely that the Management Committee would have sanctioned the letter to S's mother warning her that she would not be allowed to visit if her behaviour did not improve.

ix. The contemporary notes by Dr. Harfst and the nursing staff, and Dr. Harfst's evidence about their dealings with S's mother, reveal their determination not to hold out any olive branch to her. Dr. Harfst and the nursing staff were supporting each other in a hostile combination against her. Dr. Harfst should have been leading the staff away from retaliatory measures, not lending them support. It may well be that they were all convinced that they were right and that what they were doing was in the best interests of all the patients and staff in Cypress. But they were wrong, and their weapons were indignity and humiliation. Frustration, stress, lack of support and lack of guidance all played their part.

x. But for the sustained campaign by S's mother he would not have been moved out of Cypress Villa in November 1969 or to another hospital in January 1970, and Cypress Villa would not have been closed as a security villa at that time.

1969-1972. Cypress as a Ward for Disturbed Patients

292. On 3 December 1969 the Secretary of the Board sent an "Authority for Action" to Dr. Ramsay:

1. " That Cypress Ward . . . should cease to function as a unit for patients requiring a high degree of security.
2. That the admission policy regarding this unit should be brought into line with that pertaining for the rest of the South Ockendon Group.
3. That the Senior Administrative Medical Officer report again in two months' time on the future use of the facilities of the unit ".

293. On 23 December 1969 Dr. Ramsay wrote to the Department of Health and Social Security " The Board have already discussed the problems arising in Cypress Ward and would wish to change its use from a security unit to a more open ward so that it might give some relief to the grave overcrowding of South Ockendon Hospital. This would not preclude a degree of security, but only for those suitable for treatment within the general ambience of the hospital ".

294. Minute 5104 of the Hospital Management Committee meeting held on 2 January 1970 records that the Committee " approved the decision that Cypress Villa should no longer exist as a security unit. This was now operating as an open ward and there was a slight easement of the overcrowding ".

295. Dr. Ramsay reported to the Board's Finance and General Purposes Committee on 21 January 1970 that its earlier decision " that the admission policy of the unit should be brought into line with that pertaining for the rest of the Group " had been implemented by the Hospital Management Committee and that the Board's Advisory Committee in Psychiatry had agreed with that action.

296. How had these decisions been translated into action? Dr. Harfst told us that he had attended the meeting of the Advisory Committee and that it had been decided that Cypress should be used for disturbed and difficult patients from elsewhere in the hospital. It was not, so far as we could ascertain, reported to the Management Committee that Cypress was to be used for such patients. The decision as to which patients should be moved was taken by Dr. Harfst after discussion with Dr. Dutton. Two or three were discharged. The rest were transferred to other villas in the hospital, the vacancies being created by the transfer of disturbed patients from Beech to Cypress.

297. Quite clearly the use of Cypress was not changing from a security unit to an ordinary open villa as recorded in the Management Committee minutes. It was essential that a clear policy should be laid down for the villa and explained to the staff. Dr. Harfst was asked " what steps did you take to impress on the nursing staff and junior medical staff that the idea of Cypress being security-minded was to be a thing of the past?" A. " I did not take any. I did not think it was necessary. It was quite obvious to everyone, and everyone was familiar with the arrangement on other wards, particularly on Beech, and it was simply a transfer of that function ".

298. The nature of the change, however, was not clear to the staff. There is an entry for 30 December 1969 in the Charge Nurses' Handover Book " Re Dr. Harfst's visit on Saturday: he says Cypress will no longer be a maximum security ward and that he is going to discharge or transfer to other wards as many patients as possible. They will be replaced by disturbed patients from Beech and Limes. He says restrictions can be relaxed on the ward and all internal doors need not be kept locked. It all seems a bit vague just now and there are no written instructions ". Since that time the records show that Dr. Harfst has visited Cypress Villa less than once a fortnight, although he says that his visits have not always been recorded. In our view the policy should have been worked out by a Hospital Multi-disciplinary Team and translated into action in unit multi-disciplinary meetings.

John Meter

299. One of the disturbed patients transferred from another part of the hospital to Cypress Ward in December 1969 was a psychotic boy, John Meter, who at this time was 14 years old.

300. John's early development was reported to be normal, but at the age of two and a half his progress became arrested and since then he has presented a severe and persistent behaviour problem and has proved ineducable. He attended a training centre for half-days for several years but was a very disturbing influence and a danger to the other children because of his biting habits. Between 1965 and 1968 he was admitted to South Ockendon Hospital several times for short-term care. Unsuccessful attempts were made to place him in some other hospital. He was admitted to a Rudolf Steiner school but had to leave after one term. The Superintendent of the school reported " John continues to require the complete attention of one person at all times and has begun to attack even the most helpless children ". He was admitted as an inpatient to South Ockendon Hospital in May 1968 and spent some time in Pines Ward before being transferred to Cypress Ward in December 1969. In July 1969 Dr. Dutton's Registrar

77

wrote to Mrs. Meter asking her to sign an authority for John to be given Electro Convulsive Therapy. He wrote " His condition is not too bad at present but is deteriorating ".

301. Until the death of his father in September 1971 John was taken home each weekend. After that Mrs. Meter was unable to take him home. The first time she visited him without taking him home he kept running back to the side room. From that time on his condition deteriorated further: he became more withdrawn and would not stay in the day room with her but went back to the side room. He refused to wear clothes from about November 1971. Early in 1972 Mrs. Meter gave up her job and visited her son almost daily, at first for four hours a day and later for one hour.

302. In May 1972 John was sent to Oxford for an independent re-assessment. He was admitted to an adult psychiatric ward at the Warneford Hospital. A special nurse was allocated to his care throughout the day shifts and spent a great portion of his time dealing with John. John returned to South Ockendon Hospital a month later on 5 June, showing some small improvement. From about the end of July, his mother occasionally succeeded in persuading him to put on clothes for an hour or so and to go for a walk in the grounds of the hospital.

303. Mrs. Meter gave evidence to us and also allowed us to see a diary which she kept of her visits to John between 16 April 1972 and 5 July 1972. She was a candid and sincere witness who showed a driving desire to help her son, however hopeless the quest might sometimes seem. Her diary gave a day-by-day account of the small events which made up John's life in Cypress Villa, and of her own reactions of hope or anxiety to John's behaviour, and of gratitude or resentment towards the various nurses.

304. Mrs. Meter had two main complaints:—
   i. That South Ockendon Hospital was not a suitable hospital for providing the care needed by John.
   ii. That the standard of care given in Cypress Villa caused John's condition to deteriorate.

Suitability of South Ockendon Hospital for the care of John

305. From the outset Dr. Dutton held the firm view, which he did not withhold from Mrs. Meter, that South Ockendon Hospital was unsuitable for John and that he would deteriorate because of the lack of proper facilities. In April 1965 he diagnosed juvenile psychosis and in a report of 4 April of that year he wrote " I do not think it will be in the boy's best interests to be admitted to a ward in this hospital where he would be faced with an environment which could only do harm ". He made strenuous efforts to avoid having to take such a hazardous step. In October 1965 he tried without success to arrange for John's admission to Borocourt Hospital. On 25 October he wrote to Dr. O'Gorman describing John as " to my way of thinking an undoubtedly autistic child rather than a mentally retarded boy, and I must admit my sympathies are on her (the mother's) side as we have no facilities for dealing with these disturbed children other than blotting them out with drugs ".

306. In May 1966 Dr. O'Gorman saw John as an outpatient. He wrote to Dr. Dutton on 11 May " There is nothing I can tell you about his clinical

condition that you do not know already. He shows most of the typical autistic features . . . As to disposal I am quite sure this boy ought to be in hospital, and although he is psychotic, he is mentally subnormal just as much as if he were suffering from epiloia. I would therefore be inclined to admit him to South Ockendon, if only as a means of helping the family, for the mother's life must be an awful misery ".

307. On 23 November 1966 Mrs. Meter wrote to Dr. Dutton to thank him for his efforts. She went on " Although the prospects for John do not appear too good at the moment, I do not see why I should go against your advice and send John to South Ockendon. I doubt if I shall get anywhere, but I am going to write to my M.P. and a few others, and strongly protest about the lack of suitable care for children like John in this area. It is shameful in this day and age that these poor children continue to be left out in the cold ".

308. Mrs. Meter wrote to Mr. Driberg M.P. and since that time he has done all he can to help Mrs. Meter. He visited John in hospital and gave evidence to us of the conditions he found.

309. Dr. Harfst, the consultant psychiatrist for Pines and Cypress Villas, reported in April 1969 that John was suffering from autistic features attendant upon a juvenile psychosis, and that in view of his disturbed state and aggression no environment other than a psychiatric hospital would be able to contain him.

310. We have already stated that John was admitted to South Ockendon as a long-stay patient in May 1968 and that by July 1969 the deterioration antici- pated by Dr. Dutton was already taking place. In November 1969 Mrs. Meter found John confined to a side room in Pines Villa without a bed and with the windows wholly covered by shutters. He had a mattress on the floor. The ex- planation put forward was that he had broken his bed and that it could not be repaired until after the weekend. The shutters were said to be necessary in order to prevent escape. A regime should not have been tolerated in which it was considered necessary to deprive a patient of daylight for part of a day, let alone days on end.

311. Dr. O'Gorman saw John again in April 1972 and discussed his case at length in a letter to Dr. Harfst. He concluded that " John is a very severe nursing problem indeed " and that he could not do more for him at Borocourt Hospital than could be done at South Ockendon Hospital, " indeed I think perhaps we could do less since our nurse to patient ratio on similar wards is worse than yours ". The extent of the problem as seen from the nursing staff's point of view was vividly described by Mr. Hubbard in a document dated 14 April 1972 which is set out in Appendix 6.

312. In May 1972 John was transferred to Warneford Hospital, Oxford, for comprehensive assessment taking about a month. We were supplied with a copy of the assessment made jointly by Dr. Stores and Dr. Taylor who also gave evidence before us. They had found evidence of brain damage which in their opinion made it inappropriate for John to be considered as a case of true autism, and concluded that long term placement in a subnormality hospital was ap- propriate. Whilst at Warneford, John " remained naked throughout his stay, repeatedly he would grunt or mutter or scream in a high-pitched manner when frustrated, frightened or enraged, and he bit other people or his own forearm in similar circumstances. In these respects there was no convincing change during

his stay, or at least not a consistent change. Initially he confined himself to his room . . . preferred his own door closed and preferred people not to enter the room, but as time went on he became more interested in the activities outside his own room and insisted on the door remaining open. On the other hand, he insisted on other doors in the ward being closed ". At first he soiled the floor, walls and door but later, with encouragement, he used a urinal in his room and used the W.C. properly though his performance was variable. He was intolerant of clothes, and of the locker, the bed and the mattress in his room and he was destructive.

313. Dr. Stores could not quote the staffing ratios on the ward, but said that it was possible for one member of the nursing staff to be allocated to manage John's case almost full-time at any one time and this was how the encouragement was given. He said " At South Ockendon Hospital there was no prospect of doing anything more for this patient than was done because they were unable to allocate to him one member of the staff full-time which really was necessary to make any progress ". Dr. Taylor explained that his hospital was not having to care for this patient for very long, and this affected both the staff's attitude of mind and the ability of the hospital to bring great resources to bear upon the problem. Asked what would be the ideal answer to the long term placement of John Meter he replied: " An ideal answer would require not only that we had very large resources of money available to spend in this way, and that that was thought a reasonable and wise thing to do with our resources; and then that we found the personnel who were prepared to spend their lives doing this sort of work. Granted both of those, then there could be establishments which could be set up which could look after patients like John Meter on a long term basis. Failing that we have to make what we can with what resources are made available to us and with what humanity we can find ". He agreed that in practice the answer was that such patients should have as many qualified staff as possible constantly looking after them, so that the personal relationship which Warneford Hospital staff were able to establish with John could as nearly as possible be achieved elsewhere.

The standard of care of John Meter in Cypress Villa

314. There was little dispute between Mrs. Meter and the hospital staff over matters of fact; the difference of view lay in the reason for the conditions and the possibility of curing them. It was accepted by all parties that during the first six months in Cypress Ward John spent most of his time in a side room and that the conditions in the side room were as Mrs. Meter described them. John was naked and the room was unfurnished except for a mattress on the floor; there were often faeces and urine on the floor. There was no bell and he had to bang on the door to attract attention. When Mrs. Meter arrived on a visit she frequently cleaned the floor and threw out the mattress. She complained that the faeces were sometimes solid, suggesting that they had been there some time.

315. Mr. Lewis, who was a charge nurse in Cypress Villa for part of this period, described the difficulties of managing John. During his disturbed periods it was necessary for him to be locked in the side room to prevent biting attacks on other patients and staff. When less disturbed, he still preferred to stay in the side room and was reluctant to leave it. The nursing staff made constant attempts to dress him, helped sometimes by his mother, but without success. He rejected a bed completely until after his return from Warneford Hospital. This was demon-

strated to Mrs. Meter on one of her visits. Many mattresses were destroyed by John and different types were tried. Those with a plastic mattress cover had to be removed because he would get between the cover and the mattress, and the nurses feared he might be asphyxiated. A mattress covered with plasticised ticking was briefly satisfactory, but then John tore off the outer cover and lay on the ticking which soon became soiled and had to be destroyed. A foam rubber type with a nylon cover was also tried, but John tore off the cover and lay on the foam rubber. For a long period John got through an average of two mattresses a week, sometimes two mattresses in a day. Although John was physically capable of being continent, he began to show bizarre behaviour with regard to his excrement when his general behaviour deteriorated and he had to spend more time in the side room. He would be taken to the lavatory " and as soon as he had got back into the room he would open his bowels on the floor and tread it on the floor, smear it on his body, the walls and the windows ". Often he deliberately held his urine when at the lavatory and then urinated on the floor as soon as he was taken back to the side room. We are unable to assess the extent to which this behaviour was caused or aggravated by the fact that John could not leave the side room and go to the lavatory when he wanted. Mr. Lewis said that when he was in charge John was taken out of his side room every day after his breakfast, that attempts were made to dress him, and that the orderly cleaned out the side room. He said that although John could not himself get out of the side room he was frequently taken to the lavatory except when Mrs. Meter was coming when they left it to her to take him.

316. Mrs. Meter complained particularly about an occasion in January 1972 when she managed to dress John and take him to a hospital party but had to take him straight back again as he would not stay. On return to the side room she found that the mattress was so filthy it was stuck to the floor and the faeces looked as though it had been there for at least two days. " I had to get several buckets of water and throw them on the floor and let the floor soak before I could shift it off the floor. It was also on the windows and doors ". Mr. Lewis' explanation was that the entire staff had been engaged in dressing all the patients in their best clothes for the party and that was why John's room had been allowed to get into a dirty condition.

317. Mrs. Meter thought that if the side room door could be opened from the inside John would go to the lavatory instead of soiling his room. Mr. Lewis said to us " My attitude was always to try and keep him out of the side room as far as possible, but on the few occasions we wanted him in the side room we wanted him to stay there ". When asked why the door could not have a handle on both sides and the room be locked when necessary he frankly said " it never entered my head ". Mrs. Meter said she had discussed this with another nurse in July 1972 and he had promised to see if he could get something done about it, but the position was still unchanged up to 17 September.

318. Mrs. Meter complained several times that John was cold. Mr. Lewis admitted that the heating might be inadequate when it first came on but generally it was good and " the temperature in Cypress Villa at times is almost unbearable ". He said that the windows were opened to let fresh air in and that John was warmer running round in the corridor which was lined with radiators than he would be static in the side room. He strongly disagreed with Mrs. Meter's habit of putting John back into the side room.

319. Mr. Blackburn, a young psychologist on the staff of the hospital, suggested a course of behaviour therapy to try to persuade John to wear clothes. If he put on a garment he would be given food, but, if he refused, food would be withheld for up to three days. The experiment failed. It was only tried for five weeks and Mr. Blackburn then agreed to it being stopped without coming to see what the problems were or whether modifications could be made.

320. Dr. Harfst said that John was too disturbed to mix with work groups as he was liable to attack other patients. His powers of concentration were very poor. In order to receive training he would need continuous individual attention and this was beyond the scope or resources of South Ockendon Hospital. Mr. Lewis said that when he suggested to Mrs. Meter that she should help to look after John in Cypress Villa he had thought she had insight into the type of training and encouragement he needed and that she would have the drive, tolerance and patience to persist with it. He was disappointed. " She would sit outside the side room on a chair with an ashtray beside her and occasionally lock in at him ". Asked what had been done to show her how to go about the job he replied " You could not explain to Mrs. Meter. I just was unable to get through to her at this stage ". We do not accept this. Mr. Lewis' real difficulty was that he did not know how to make any progress with John, and this, coupled with shortage of time and lack of guidance on how best to help her, led him to leave her too much on her own. We have no doubt that he wanted to help and we are sure that he would have done if he had known how to set about it.

321. Apart from nursing care and treatment, John has received treatment with a variety of drugs. He has also in the past received courses of Electro-Convulsive Therapy, which initially resulted in improvement although this was followed by relapse. Mrs. Meter was unwilling for him to receive this form of treatment again as she believed that any good effects were shortlived and were outweighted by the distress to John of being held down by nurses. She felt that Electro-Convulsive Therapy was used as an emergency measure to quieten John down, rather than as part of a long term treatment plan. In our view she was right. In March 1972, her solicitor sent a letter to Dr. Harfst asking for an assurance that this form of treatment would not be given again without her consent, and following this she had a discussion with Dr. Harfst in which she understood him to present her with three alternatives: either to have John at home, or to let him have Electro-Convulsive Therapy, or to see him sent to Rampton. She replied that she would rather struggle with John at home than send him to Rampton. Dr. Harfst in evidence agreed that he was a bit annoyed to receive a letter from the solicitor after Mrs. Meter had agreed to a further course of Electro-Convulsive Therapy and arangements had been made for it. He said that he was quite sure she could not manage John at home and that he had it in mind that a relatively short stay at Rampton, where there was a greater concentration of staff, might effect an improvement which could then be maintained at South Ockendon. Whatever Dr. Harfst intended to convey, we are satisfied that Mrs. Meter understood that he was threatening to send John to Rampton Special Hospital for an indefinite period unless she was more co-operative. This episode concluded with a letter from Dr. Harfst to the solicitor in which he explained that her consent for Electro-Convulsive Therapy was unnecessary as John had reached the age of 16 and he refused to give the undertaking requested, but stated that if Mrs. Meter was unhappy about this form of treatment he would not " make a big

issue of it ". No further course of this treatment has in fact been given. In our view Dr. Harfst would have been more persistent but for the solicitor's letters.

322. Dr. Harfst said in evidence that on John's return from Oxford he had changed his drug treatment. He removed all drugs except one (a tranquillising drug) and increased the dosage of this one. Although this change coincided with John's improvement, Dr. Harfst did not think it could all be attributed to the drug. The hospital staff were hard at work trying to build on the improvement, but he had grave fears that there would be a relapse.

Conclusions

323.
    i. South Ockendon Hospital was the only residential accommodation available and willing to take John Meter. It was suitable only in the very limited sense that it was impossible for John to remain at home any longer and there was nowhere else for him to go.

    ii. It is clear that John Meter presents a very difficult management problem, and we commend the staff at South Ockendon Hospital for their perseverance in caring for him and in seeking new ways to improve his condition.

    iii. We accept Mrs. Meter's evidence that the standard of care has too often been too low, as regards the cleanliness, smell, heating and ventilation of the side room. We recommend that the handle and lock of the side room door should be altered so that John can be free to leave the room at will except when his condition is such that he needs to be locked in for his own safety or for the safety of others. Renewed efforts should be made to encourage him to use the lavatory. Means should be found of improving the ventilation and the occasional inadequacy of the heating of the side room.

    iv. The hospital staff appear to have tried all the usual methods of medical treatment for John's condition, which is one for which there is as yet no known cure. The friction over Dr. Harfst's proposal to repeat Electro-Convulsive Therapy treatment in March 1972 was another example of his inability to communicate in an understanding and friendly way with the concerned mother of a patient.

    v. We consider that the experiment in behaviour therapy was not persisted in long enough to judge whether it could prove valuable, and that the psychologist should have visited the ward to check on the progress being made before agreeing to the abandonment of the programme.

    vi. Early in 1972 Mrs. Meter was willing to spend several hours a day at the hospital to help with the care of her son but she found difficulty in coping with him and received little help from the staff. We have the impression that the staff were not unhappy to see her finding the same difficulties as they had met. This was unfortunate. Much might have been achieved with an extra person to look after John if she had been offered and had been willing to receive help and guidance in playing with him and trying to modify his behaviour. There may still in the future be the possibility of such an experiment if both Mrs. Meter and the hospital staff are willing to regard her as a voluntary, unqualified, but experienced, member of the team looking after John.

vii. We accept the expert evidence that a subnormality hospital such as South Ockendon Hospital is at present more suitable than other places to care for John Meter. John Meter unfortunately is not unique. We very much hope that resources will soon be made available so that patients like him can be given the kind of care they need. This means initially a period of intensive care, with one nurse staying with the patient throughout the day and attempting to alleviate his condition so that he may become less dependent. Such care requires the equivalent of about three whole-time nurses for each patient in order to allow for weekends, holidays and so on, and we realise the difficulty of providing this even for a short term whilst the shortage of nurses continues. In our view the provision of adequate facilities and supporting staff would help recruitment. In the meantime John Meter will have to continue at South Ockendon Hospital where the staff/patient ratio, although above the national average for subnormality hospitals, is far below that required by such patients. We believe that all concerned with John's care will do their best in these difficult circumstances. We recommend that as many nurses as is reasonably possible should be allocated to the care of disturbed patients like John, and that they should be cared for in smaller groups.

Allegations of Violence in Cypress during 1972

Patient U

324. On 21 April 1972 a patient alleged that on the previous day a coloured nurse in Cypress had struck a patient in the mouth and had struck another across the buttock with a belt. Prompt action was taken and the patients were examined. The patient who was alleged to have been struck in the mouth had a slight laceration inside the mouth. The other one had no marks. When Mr. Hardas, the charge nurse, was asking other staff whether they had witnessed these alleged assaults Mr. Prentis, a Nursing Assistant, reported that he had seen Mr. Dookhith, a coloured pupil nurse, strike a patient, U, on the previous afternoon.

325. All these matters were referred to the police who after full investigation decided to take no action.

326. In view of the lapse of three months before our Committee could hear evidence we did not enquire into those allegations of assault which depended entirely on the evidence of the patients. We did not consider that we would be able to reach any sure conclusion. We did however hear evidence about the alleged assault on U.

327. Mr. Prentis said that he was in the television lounge at about 5.00 p.m. with Mr. Dookhith and a number of patients. Mr. Dookhith and U were sitting in chairs close to one another. Suddenly without any warning or provocation U struck Mr. Dookhith on his back with the flat of the hand. Mr. Dookhith then appeared to lose his temper and pulled U out of his chair and appeared to knee him in the face. He then pulled U into the day room. There U was either pushed or fell to the floor and Mr. Dookhith kicked him two or three times in the region of the chest. He then took U to the toilet area where Mr. Prentis

heard him screaming and shouting. He was asked if he said anything to Mr. Dookhith and he replied " Not at the time. It is very awkward. I did not know him. When someone is above you it is very awkward to say anything ". Later he was asked why he did not complain to the charge nurse at once. He said "Well, you see, in cases like that you are always tempted not to say anything. It is a horrible thing to say, but it is true, because you don't want trouble. I admit I would not have said anything if I had not been asked by the charge nurse ".

328. Mr. Dookhith agreed that he had been slapped on the back by U and that he had then seen that he was mumbling and spitting. He therefore decided to take him to the toilet area in case he injured the other patients. He said that he got up and approached U who was still sitting in his chair, and that U then started to get up and he got hold of his hands. He said that he was at no time angry. He took U to the toilet area where he kicked out at the wall but quickly quietened down.

329. Two other nurses who were on duty in the villa at the time said that they saw nothing of the incident and were probably out of the room when it occurred. Dr. Benton examined U at 6.30 p.m. on 21 April and again on the 22nd but found no marks.

Conclusion

330. We are satisfied that Mr. Dookith lost his temper with U, pulled him roughly from his chair and then kneed him. We are not able to say precisely where, or with what force, the knee made contact with U. We are further satisfied that while U was dragged through the day room he either fell or was pushed and that Mr. Dookhith kicked him two or three times in the region of the chest. We are not satisfied that any of the blows were so hard that they must have left marks which would have been visible 25 hours later at the time of Dr. Benton's examination.

Patient PP

331. The mother of two sons PP and NN, both of whom are patients in Cypress, told us that PP had complained to her in June 1972 that he had been hit frequently. He had also complained to her that he had been given an injection with a blunt needle by a charge nurse, Mr. D. J. Schreeche-Powell.

332. Mr. Schreeche-Powell explained that PP was receiving injections of Modecate. This is a thick substance and the injection of it may cause some pain even with a sharp needle. We are satisfied that a blunt needle was not used. The allegations of violence were vague and we did not feel that we would be able to make any firm finding and therefore investigated them no further.

An incident witnessed by Mrs. Meter

333. Mrs. Meter whose son is a patient in Cypress Villa visited him on 8 June 1972. She was going down the corridor at bath time in order to fetch her son a blanket when she heard squealing and screaming round the corner. She said that as she turned the corner she saw a student nurse, Mr. Acero, holding one of eight or nine naked patients against the wall and punching him on the left ear. As she reached him he stopped and looked at her and smiled. Mrs. Meter immediately reported what she had seen to the charge nurse.

334. Mr. Acero said Mrs. Meter had been mistaken in what she thought she had seen. He explained the patient had been incontinent and he had taken him to the toilet area to change his clothes. When he was undressed he ran away down the passage banging his face with his left hand. Mr. Acero said he followed him and caught hold of the left wrist to prevent him hurting himself. He said that the patient was strong and that he had difficulty in restraining him. He denied that he had struck him, or that his hand was anywhere near the patient's head. Mr. Acero's evidence was supported by Mr. Fokheer, a pupil nurse.

335. We have no doubt that Mrs. Meter was a wholly honest witness: nevertheless we think there was just room for her to have made an honest mistake as to what was happening. We are satisfied that Mr. Acero was using considerably more force than he accepts, and more than he need have done, to control the patient, but we are not satisfied that he deliberately punched him on the ear.

336. These episodes lead us to the view that too much force is not infrequently used to control violent or disobedient patients in Cypress Villa.

Cypress Villa Today

337. We went round Cypress Villa on 31 July and 28 September 1972. It is a bleak unhomely building with severe spartanly furnished rooms. On our first visit all internal doors were unlocked to let us through and then locked behind us. One of our members got separated from the rest of us by a locked door. At lunch time a door was unlocked and the patients surged through to their food. Between our first and second visits a number of questions were asked about locked doors, and on our second visit we were not surprised to find the internal doors were unlocked. But the nurse, who took us round, on several occasions put out the key in his hand to unlock the door ahead and had to withdraw it when he remembered that there was no need. We left satisfied that there was an excessive use of locked doors and that Cypress had only ceased to be a security unit in name. On our second visit there were a number of patients sitting about doing nothing or sleeping. Two nurses who had only started work in the villa a few days earlier were standing about. There was no sign of occupation or the means of occupation.

338. We asked Dr. Harfst about the locking of doors.

Q. " How are you running the unit at the present moment? " A. " I am trying to run it just as any other ward in the hospital. I do not regard it as being any different from the other wards. It contains patients who were on the other wards, and although it has a concentration of disturbed patients it is not such a concentration, and they are under more ideal conditions than the patients were on Beech. I would not say that there was any aspect of security left in the situation . . . "

Q. " What about locked doors inside the villa now? " A. " I have not made any rules about locking the doors. Nursing staff use their own initiative as they would in any other wards, all of which have locks. At least, I think they all have locks on the doors. Locked doors are used. The structure of the building is such that it allows various compartments to be used for different kinds of patients, and it controls the movement of patients. I think nursing staff use these and use locked doors to control patients as a way for compensating for the shortage of staff ".

Q. " . . . Do you think there is any danger of that initiative being perhaps used overmuch in the direction of locking doors to compensate for staff shortage? " A. " Yes, I think there is a danger there, but I had not noticed that it is in fact being abused ".

Q. " . . . Do you think it is something that could require rather more investigation? " A. " I think it is certainly not true that there are no locked doors in Cypress, and I am aware that there are. I have not been myself worried by misuse of locked doors in the ward ".

Q. " You say you have not given any instructions to staff about locked doors. What sort of guidance have you given to them about the circumstances in which locked internal doors should be used as a kind of substitute for staff shortage? " A. " I have not given them any ".

Q. " It is really left to the discretion of the individual charge nurse? It may vary from one to the other? " A. " Yes ".

Q. "Do you think that is really satisfactory? " A. " I do not think it is, but then I do not really know what instructions I could give. It is a thing which comes up for discussion every now and then in the handling of individual patients . . . I do not think that I could really lay down instructions on the subject. It is one thing I do not like doing anyway, giving instructions to nursing staff about things which I regard anyway as matters for their discretion ".

339. Dr. Harfst went on to agree that the degree to which locked doors should be used as a substitute for staff was more a matter of policy than discretion, but said that he had not seen anything in Cypress which made him want to state a policy about it. He knew of no hospital policy about the locking of internal doors and thought that it was left to the discretion of the staff in each villa.

340. We are satisfied that the side rooms continued to be used for punishment purposes from time to time. Dr. Harfst approves of such use although he prefers the expression " education ". He says that he would not prescribe a set term of seclusion and would take steps to prevent this being done. We cannot accept that this was his view in 1970. On 4 August that year the clinical records of patient SS show that he was ordered to be confined to a side room for one week for becoming aggressive and hitting out at staff members. It was recorded that he was to be seen by Dr. Harfst who interviewed him on 17 August and made the next entry on the clinical record. This makes it clear that the interview was about the behaviour for which he had been confined for one week. In October 1970 there is another entry by Dr. Benton ordering that the same patient be confined to a side room for one week for attacking a member of the staff.

341. We have already said that Dr. Dutton told us that he regards the Cypress regime as too rigid, but that this is not something that he would bring up for discussion at the Medical Executive Committee. There was no evidence that he had discussed his present doubts about Cypress with anybody.

Conclusions

342. The events and attitudes which we have just set out are not acceptable to us. Dr. Dutton, although he claims to have been unhappy about the regime, had done nothing about it because it lay within the boundaries of Dr. Harfst's

clinical autonomy. Dr. Harfst has failed to give direction and guidance in a field where direction and guidance were urgently needed. The inadequate numbers of staff have done their best in most instances, but inevitably, without proper guidance, they have carried on the locked door tradition. The patients have suffered as a result.

343. The patients, staffing and aims of this villa must be urgently reviewed.

CHAPTER VI

WILLOWS VILLA

344. We now turn to the events which led directly to the setting up of this inquiry. They took place in Willows Villa during December 1971 and January and February 1972. At the beginning of that period it was the home of 48 sub-normal and severely subnormal men. The majority were aged between forty and sixty years, but the range of ages started below thirty and extended to about seventy. Some were overactive while others were prematurely senile and regarded as geriatric patients by some staff. The consultant responsible for the villa was Dr. Harfst. Mr. Large was one of the two charge nurses working in it by day.

345. On 6 December Mrs. Youell, a State Enrolled Nurse, commenced a spell of night duty on Willows. Between that date and 17 February 1972 seven of the patients died, one of them as a result of severe internal bruising. On 17 February Mrs. Youell resigned from the staff of the hospital and made the written allegations in Appendix 7 about the standard of care in the villa. These eventually resulted in this inquiry. Explaining her resignation to us she said " I grew very attached to certain patients that died, and seeing the way they died it just put me off nursing. I said I would never go back again; I just re-signed. But I felt something should be done for the remaining patients, or some attention should be drawn to this ward. That is all I wanted ". In another part of her evidence she said that it was the fact that she was getting nowhere that made her resign. " It was getting worse on Willows. The patients appeared to be dying one after the other. It was not that they were dying. I am not trying to be God, I firmly believe that when your time is up, it is up. But it is how they went, how they were treated when they were dying or sick. This is what I am complaining about ".

346. We propose, first, to make an assessment of Mrs. Youell's personality and capabilities as a nurse and to compare it with that of Mr. Large and Mr. Turkington, the two charge nurses. We will then consider her complaints relating to :
a. the care of patients
b. administrative matters,
and, having set out our findings, we shall examine how Mrs. Youell's complaints were received and dealt with.

347. In a further section we shall consider allegations of unkind treatment of patients made by Mrs. Woods, a pupil nurse.

Assessment of Mrs. Youell

348. Mrs. Youell has been engaged in nursing for about 20 years in Ireland and England. Her experience includes the nursing of acute, psychiatric and geriatric patients and also patients suffering from tuberculosis.

349. She started as a cadet nurse in Ireland and then came to England. During her third year of training, when she was engaged in acute psychiatric

nursing, her brother died and she had to return to her family in Ireland. She subsequently married and did not complete the course. She started work at South Ockendon Hospital in about 1961 and became a State Enrolled Nurse in 1968. She has six children, four of whom have been born while she has been working at South Ockendon. On each occasion she has had three months' " maternity leave ". The last child was born in 1969. Mrs. Youell's husband also worked in the hospital for about the same period. He has qualified in the nursing of subnormal patients and has been a charge nurse for about seven years.

350. In the course of her eleven years at the hospital Mrs. Youell worked in Limes, Pines, Hawthorns and Briars Villas and the Gloucester Clinic. She had spent the $1\frac{1}{2}$ years before December 1971 working in Briars, apart from a short period of under a month in Willows earlier in 1971. She was moved from Briars to Willows in December 1971 because her husband was also working in Briars at that time, and this on occasions caused difficulty with other staff.

351. Mr. Hubbard, Mr. Macdonald, Mr. Margan, Mr. Mitra, Mr. Large and Mr. Turkington all regarded Mrs. Youell as a very good and conscientious nurse. There seemed to be general agreement, however, that during the last few months of her service at the hospital she became increasingly anxious and appeared to be under some strain, although this did not affect her work. She had taken Mogadon for about two years as she had difficulty in sleeping following her father's death. Early in 1971 she was treated for an ulcer, and in June 1971 her gall bladder was removed. Towards the end of 1971, while she was still working in Briars, she commenced to suffer from anxiety and Valium was prescribed. A short trial period on Librium was not a success.

352. We considered that Mrs. Youell was a very good and very conscientious nurse right up to the time of her resignation. She is an attractive and sensitive woman whose standards were higher than those she found in Willows. She suffered from anxiety which was aggravated by her inability to get the standard of care in Willows improved. One witness was called before us who said that on one evening when Mrs. Youell came on duty she was under the influence of drugs. We rejected this evidence which was denied by another witness.

Assessment of Mr Large

353. Mr. Large entered nursing in 1962. We are satisfied that he wished to improve the conditions in which his subnormal patients lived. He spent some of his off duty hours doing things for them. He was aware of the needs of his patients but, in our view, easily became dissatisfied and discouraged. His attitude then became surly.

354. Between 1962 and March 1967 Mr. Large spent the greater part of his time at Darenth Park Hospital, commencing as a student nurse and finishing as a staff nurse. He then spent some months at the Ida Darwin Hospital as a staff nurse. At both hospitals he acted as a charge nurse at times. He came to South Ockendon Hospital as a charge nurse in the autumn of 1967. The reference from the Principal Nursing Officer of the Ida Darwin Hospital, although saying that Mr. Large was of quiet disposition and of good character and was suitable for employment as a charge nurse, went on to add " [it] appears to me that he is unable to settle for long. . . . He was a little disappointed that he was not promoted recently ". The reference from the Deputy Medical Superintendent

at Darenth Park said he had discharged his nursing and administrative duties as an Acting Charge Nurse " quite well ". The Chief Male Nurse at Darenth Park, however, sounded a clear warning in his reference. He described his disposition and character as " Surly. Inclined to become dissatisfied ". In answer to the question " Do you consider the applicant a suitable person to enter the employment of the Committee? " he wrote " Not as a charge nurse ".

355. Dr. Jones, who had known Mr. Large at Darenth Park, supported his application to come to South Ockendon Hospital as a charge nurse, but it is probable that the major factor in his appointment was the difficulty in obtaining staff at the hospital.

356. We called a number of witnesses before us at the request of Mr. Large. One was Mrs. Thorne whose son has been a patient in the hospital for nine years. He has been in Beech Villa since December 1971, but he spent the three years before that in Willows. Mr. Large was a charge nurse for that villa from June 1970 onwards. Mrs. Thorne is employed as a shop assistant in the hospital and has been a member of the League of Friends for nine years. We found her an impressive witness. She had a high opinion of Mr. Large but she found that the standard of care deteriorated in the villa during 1970 and 1971. She thought he was " trying too hard really. He got himself into a very distressing state—trying so hard to get some things for the patients such as clothing and what have you ". She said that his depression and frustration seemed to increase as time went by. Mr. Large told us that the events in Beech in 1968 and 1969 were a traumatic experience for him and he felt mentally and physically drained. He consulted his General Practitioner and was given tablets which he had to take for about a year. He said " I took the opinion that I would stay at my post to prove that I could do the job. I did not want people to think that I was leaving the hospital because I could not cope. I stayed to prove to myself that I could handle the job and because I like the hospital and many of the people there were very good to me and I formed many friendships there amongst the staff and patients ". He said that during his time in Willows " it became increasingly more difficult. I had to battle with things that were not tangible, things like staff morale. I mean how can you get people to do these distasteful tasks when the morale of the staff is low? This is why I did try to boost the morale of staff by not having a regimented system on the ward ".

Assessment of Mr. Turkington

357. Mr. Turkington comes from Ireland where he worked as a nursing assistant in subnormal hospitals from 1957 to 1961, in which year he started work at South Ockendon Hospital. He was promoted to Charge Nurse in about 1970 and has worked in Willows since January 1971. Mrs. Thorne thought that he required more experience before being made a charge nurse. We agree with her. He is a follower rather than a leader.

Mrs. Youell's Complaints about the Care of Patients

General

358. Mrs. Youell's complaints about the general standard of care are best expressed in her own words.

Q. " What was your immediate impression about the nursing standards on Willows . . . ? " A. " My immediate reaction was that I could not believe it. . . . I always thought that other parts of the hospital were quite high [in standard of care] for a subnormal hospital. When I went to Willows I was really distressed at what I saw ".

Q. " . . . what were the things . . . which distressed you most of all ? " A. " In their clothing and appearance, and they were forsaken-looking. The staff were looking at television, and the patients needed attention to me. Whereas in other wards there would be hustle and bustle to get the patients cared for ".

She went on to describe how their clothing appeared to be unnecessarily dirty, their nails insufficiently tended and their bodies insufficiently washed.

359. Mrs. Thorn's evidence supported Mrs. Youell. She said that when her son first went into Willows towards the end of 1968 the nursing standard was very high.

Q. " Over the years did it change in any way ? " A. " I think over the last two years it did deteriorate ".

Q. " Do you think there is any particular reason for that ? " A. " Yes I think inexperienced staff, not of [the] high standard required of nursing; and, of course, shortage of staff, sickness and staff not on duty through something or other. . .".

Q. "And how did the fall in standard show itself? " A. " Patients looked unkempt and very dismal ".

Q. " How did you observe this ? " A. " If you visit and know the patients as I know them, you only have to look at them. . .".

360. We express our conclusions on the standard of care generally at a later stage of this report. It is sufficient to say at this stage that we regard this evidence of Mrs. Youell and Mrs. Thorne as accurate and reliable.

Patient C

361. C was born in 1897 and died on 6 February 1972. He had a chronic chest condition. For some years prior to his death he was properly described as a feeble old man whose condition was gradually deteriorating.

Facts found

362. i. C collapsed on his way to bed at 9.40 p.m. on 30 January 1972. Mrs. Youell found that he was very cyanosed and could not feel his pulse. She summoned Mr. Margan, the night charge nurse, who arrived while she was giving C oxygen. This revived C sufficiently to enable them to put him to bed. Mrs. Youell commenced a Temperature, Pulse and Respiration chart for the patient.

ii. Mr. Margan asked Mrs. Youell which doctor was on call that night. When she told him that it was an outside practitioner he said that there would not be much point in calling him as he would not understand C.

iii. C became cyanosed and distressed again at 10.40 p.m. and 1.20 a.m. Oxygen was given on each occasion and at intervals up to about 3.00 a.m. Mr. Macdonald, the night superintendent, visited Willows twice during the night and on at least one of the occasions helped to administer oxygen to C. He told us " This patient was ill on several occasions prior to this, over the years. He was a very sick man actually: he had a heart condition. He had been physically ill over two or three years ".

iv. Mr. Macdonald spoke to the doctor on call on the telephone, told him of C's condition and said that he did not think he need come to see him as he had improved and had had " these turns " previously. Later in his evidence he explained that the doctor had no knowledge of C apart from what he told him on the telephone from the case notes. He went on " I was quite satisfied with his condition after the administration of oxygen. I was instructed to continue, and I told the doctor I did not think it was necessary for him to come out because this patient's condition had been deteriorating over two years: he was a very old patient ".

v. Mrs. Youell would have called a doctor if it had been in her power as " the poor old thing was coughing and holding his stomach. I was very distressed to see him ". The cough was coming up from his stomach and she had to clean lumps of mucous and phlegm out of his mouth with swabs.

vi. Mrs. Youell wrote in the ward report book that C "was up and about and looking his normal self. Had tea and was making his way to bed at 9.40 p.m. when he collapsed over empty bed. Very cyanosed, could not feel pulse. R.32, Oxygen given and pt recovered enough to be put to bed. Colour returned after 5 minutes, pulse very fast. N/C and N/S informed and visited. Pt nursed in day room because of the lights disturbing other patients and temperature in Dorm. Fluids given $++$. Pt complaining of pain in abdomen. May be due to very bad cough. Became distressed and cyanosed twice later 10.40 p.m. and 1.20 a.m. Oxygen given on both times and at intervals up to 3.00 a.m. when he appeared to be more settled. BP and TPR recorded. At time of report BP 108/68 TPR 99². 100.26 ".

vii. Mrs. Youell showed Mr. Large this report when he took over in the morning, and he said he would call the doctor. He summoned Dr. Motashaw who was a locum visiting general practitioner at the hospital and had seen C on two or three previous occasions. She knew that he had a chronic lung condition and a long standing heart condition.

viii. Dr. Motashaw saw C during the morning of 31 January. She said she did not find him " so very ill as the report suggested ". This led her to doubt the accuracy of Mrs. Youell's note. She prescribed an ordinary cough mixture. She expected a routine twice daily Temperature, Pulse and Respiration chart to be kept, but gave no instructions to the nursing staff about this. Neither did she give any instructions to the nursing staff as to whether he was to stay in bed or get up. She left it to them to decide although she would have expected him to stay in bed and be seen by the Medical Officer on the following day. Dr. Motashaw made no entry in the patient's case notes because she found " nothing very drastic wrong with the patient ", but Mr. Large entered in the ward report book that C has been "examined by MO. To commence cough linctus mane. Otherwise NAD on examination ". In the course of her evidence she was asked for what condition she had prescribed Etophylate on 7 February 1971. She said it was for C's psychological condition not for his chest condition. She was wrong in this. We accept the evidence of Dr. Benton that C had Etophylate for his bronchial spasms.

x. The cough linctus prescribed by Dr. Motashaw was not in the villa when Mrs. Youell came on duty on the evening of 31 January. Mr. Large showed her the ward report book with the entry made by him. When Mrs. Youell expressed surprise he said " if the doctor finds nothing wrong why should I worry? " He showed Mrs. Youell that he had moved C's bed to a position next to a radiator near the night post in order to make observation easier and because the temperature in the ward was low. Mrs. Youell found that C was in a neglected state. He had a furred mouth and parched lips. She tended his mouth with glycerine and tried to give him a drink which he refused. There were no notes of what diet he had had, what fluids he had taken or of his condition during the day. The Temperature, Pulse and Respiration chart which she had started the previous night was in the bin. We find that Mr. Large either put it there himself or authorised someone else to do so. He told us that he could see no point in continuing the chart as Dr. Motashaw had found nothing abnormally wrong and had not told him to carry on with it.

xi. C's condition during the night of 31 January to 1 February is described by Mrs. Youell's entry in the ward book. " Had a rough night. Severe spasms of coughing. Breathing very laboured from time to time. Oxygen given to help pt when required. Refused all fluids until early morning cup of tea. TPR 99², 110, 52 at time of report ". Mr. Macdonald visited the villa at about 10.00 p.m. and asked Mrs. Youell about C. She replied expressing despair that the doctor should report that nothing abnormal was detected when the patient was ill. Mr. Macdonald felt that he must accept the result of Dr. Motashaw's examination, but he was far from happy about the condition of the patient. Mrs. Youell did not tell Mr. Macdonald that the cough linctus was not available. If he had known this he would have got some from another ward.

xii. At 6.30 a.m. Dr. Benton came to see another patient and Mrs. Youell asked her to look at C. She did so and arranged that he should enter the Gloucester Clinic later that morning.

xiii. When Mr. Large came on duty Mrs. Youell told him what had happened. He referred to Dr. Motashaw's visit on the previous day and said " What can I do? The doctors are always too busy to pay much attention to the patients ".

xiv. It was discovered in the Gloucester Clinic that C had pneumonia. He died from it on 6 February.

Comments

363. a. The doctor should have been called on the night of 30–31 January. Instead the attitude of Mr. Margan and Mr. Macdonald seems to have

been " What is the point? The doctor won't know him, he is an old man, and has been deteriorating for a long time ".

b. Dr. Motashaw was in error in deciding that there was nothing drastically wrong with C. We are satisfied that he was a very sick man when she saw him. Mrs. Youell's written report contained factual information, not expressions of opinion, and Dr. Motashaw should not have doubted its accuracy.

c. C did not receive proper nursing care during the day of 31 January. The fact that Dr. Motashaw had found nothing abnormally wrong does not excuse this.

d. Mr. Large should have continued the Temperature, Pulse and Respiration chart started by Mrs. Youell. There was no justification for its destruction.

e. Mr. Macdonald should have sent for a doctor at 10.00 p.m. on 31 January. He allowed his misgivings about C to be lulled by the knowledge that Dr. Motashaw had found nothing abnormally wrong.

Patient D

Facts found

364.   i. D fell on his way back from Industrial Therapy on 14 February 1972.

ii. Mrs. Youell was told of this fall by Mr. Bartlett, a nursing assistant, when she came on duty that evening. She found that there was no injury report made out and no entry in the ward report book. She examined D and found multiple infected skin lesions on both legs and feet.

iii. Mrs. Youell reported D's condition to Mr. Walsh the night charge nurse. He doubted whether D had fallen and thought the marks were caused by D having his shoes laced too tightly. He said that D should remain in bed and be seen in the morning.

iv. On 15 February Dr. Benton ordered bed rest for twenty-four hours and prescribed Acetrin powder for the skin lesions on both ankles.

v. The villa treatment book contained no entry regarding the application of the Acetrin powder.

Comments

365. a. An injury report should have been made out recording that the patient had fallen and that it had then been discovered that he had skin lesions on both ankles.

b. The Acetrin powder treatment should have been entered in the treatment book.

Patient E

366. E was born on 21 January 1909 and died in Willows Ward on 21 January 1972.

Facts found

367.   i. For some time before his death E had been a frail old man whose " life hung by a thread ".

ii. On 17 January E was found to be suffering from blepharitis of the right eye. Oxytetracycline was prescribed.

iii. On the morning of 18 January Mrs. Youell told Mr. Large that she thought E should remain in bed as he had a bad chest. Although she thought it would normally be better to nurse him in an upright chair in the day room, she did not consider that this was desirable at that time as part of the floor was up and it would have been necessary to take E out of the building and in at another door. In the evening she found that he was up in his wheelchair in the day room.

iv. E liked to be up in his wheelchair in the company of other people. If he wanted to go to bed he would either say so or go of his own accord.

v. During the night of 20–21 January Dr. Benton was called to see E and found him looking " very dehydrated and frail ". He had a temperature of 100 and a very poor and variable pulse. He complained of a sore throat and cough. There were generalised harsh breathing sounds but reasonable air entry. He died at 7.20 a.m.

vi. It is not known whether E was up by day on 19 or 20 January.

Comment

368. No positive decision was taken as to whether to get E up or leave him in bed. The decision was left to the patient. There was no indication that he had received any extra attention or small comforts. The fact that he was dehydrated on 20 January indicates that he had received insufficient fluids. There was a negative approach to the care of this very frail elderly patient which cast upon him the burden of taking the decisions and asking for comforts. It was an unacceptably low standard of care which we regard as typical of that provided generally in Willows at that time.

Patient F

Facts found

369. i. At about 6.30 p.m. on 31 January 1972 F, who was then 58 years old, fell over in the toilet area. Mr. Bartlett saw that he was unable to get up and went to his assistance. With the help of Mr. Charnier and another nurse they lifted him into a wheelchair and took him to his bed. F did not appear to be in pain. Mr. Bartlett had never heard him speak. It is probable, but not certain, that Mr. Charnier put a bandage round the left leg. Mr. Bartlett or Mr. Charnier asked Mr. Large to come and look at F and he did so. We reject Mr. Large's evidence that he rotated both legs. If he had done so the patient's reactions must have made him aware that he was suffering real pain.

ii. Mr. Large made out no injury report and made no entry in the ward report book. He did not tell Mrs. Youell of the fall when she came on duty that night. We reject Mr. Large's evidence that the reason he failed to give Mrs. Youell this information was to save her from worrying. In our view he did not think the fall had caused any injury, and, therefore, did not think there was any need to inform her of it.

iii. Before Mr. Bartlett went off duty at 9.00 p.m. he told Mrs. Youell about F's fall and asked her to look at his leg. She did so. The left leg appeared very swollen and there was an abnormal rotation of the foot. She thought the leg was broken. F said he was not in pain.

iv. Mr. Margan normally visited Willows between 9.00 and 10.30 p.m. On this night he did not come on duty until about 1.00 a.m. He visited the ward about 1.30 a.m. Mrs. Youell early in this part of her evidence was sure that he had visited the ward at his normal time. She was wrong in this belief, and we consider that she may be mistaken in her recollection that she told Mr. Margan about F's leg during his visit and was told by him to report it to the charge nurse in the morning. At the time of Mr. Margan's visit F was sleeping and she may have felt that it was unnecessary to disturb him, particularly as it was a very busy night for her with many incidents occurring.

v. Mr. Macdonald went to Willows at 10.10 p.m., but this was not a normal visit by him as he was taking Mrs. Maclay round the hospital on her first night on duty under the new Salmon structure. He explained to Mrs. Youell that he could not do a normal round of the villa. Mrs. Youell did not tell him about F's leg, partly because of the nature of his visit and partly because she was busy with a lot of other incidents.

vi. At 5.00 a.m. F asked Mrs. Youell for a bottle. He normally got out of bed and went to the lavatory, so she asked if he was in pain. When he said that he was, she summoned Mr. Macdonald who came at once. He found gross displacement and thought that there was a complete fracture. He asked Mrs. Youell why she had not informed him about F and she did not reply.

vii. Mr. Macdonald summoned Dr. Benton who arrived about 5.30 a.m. She found that F's leg was externally rotated and she thought that it was fractured. She was not surprised that F had not complained to anybody. " Patients . . . often do not complain when we would expect them to ".

viii. F was transferred to the Gloucester Clinic where a fracture of the neck of the left femur was discovered. A McKee pin and plate were inserted at Orsett Hospital on 4 February and he returned to South Ockendon on 8 February.

ix. No enquiry was made by anyone in the days following as to why Mr. Large had not filled in an injury report.

Comments

370. a. Mr. Large should have noticed the abnormal rotation of the leg if he had taken sufficient trouble.

b. In any event Mr. Large should have filled in an injury report as F had fallen and had to be wheeled to his bed. Bruising might come out later.

c. Mr. Large should have informed Mrs. Youell that F had fallen, that he had been wheeled to his bed and had not since been out of it.

d. Mrs. Youell should have informed Mr. Margan or Mr. Macdonald of F's condition when they came round the villa. Her failure to do what we are confident she would normally do was caused by the combination of a particularly hectic night, Mr. Macdonald telling her at 10.10 p.m. that he could not do a normal round and Mr. Margan's failure to do his normal round early in the evening.

97

e. Mr. Large's unit nursing officer should have asked about his failure to make out an injury report or tell Mrs. Youell of F's fall.

Patient H

371. This patient suffers very badly from epilepsy. On two occasions while Mrs. Youell was on night duty he was given paraldehyde. Mrs. Youell had found from previous experience with H that paraldehyde left him unsteady on his feet and that he took about 24 hours to recover from its effect. She considered that he ought to remain in bed for that period. On at least one of the two occasions Mrs. Youell said that Mr. Large got H up in under 24 hours. She does not know at what time he got up. It may have been late in the day. In these circumstances we are unable to find whether H was fit or unfit to get up.

Patient J

Facts found

372.   i. J was born on 18 June 1904 and died on 5 April 1972. He began deteriorating noticeably in about November or December 1971. Mrs. Youell spoke to the day staff about his deterioration on several occasions.

ii. On the night of 30–31 January 1972 J's condition was as recorded by Mrs. Youell in the ward report book. " Complaining of feeling sick and pain in the region of sternum radiating around to (L) Kidney. Actal 1/1 tablet given with milk (20 oz) 9.10 p.m. which stayed down. Patient's colour became much better and he settled down. Passed continuous gas per rectum during the night. TPR 10.00 p.m. 99²–68–22, 6.00 a.m. 98²–68–20 ".

iii. When Mrs. Youell handed over to Mr. Large she showed him the report and said she thought that J should remain in bed for the day. Mr. Large said he would leave him there.

iv. Later that morning J was examined by Dr. Motashaw who found nothing abnormally wrong. It was on this morning that she also examined patient C.

v. Later that day J was got up.

Comment

373. On the evidence before us we are not satisfied that J's health suffered as a result of him getting up, but he would have been more comfortable in bed. This is another example of failure to give old and feeble patients the extra care and comforts they should have received.

Patient K

Facts found

374.   i. K was aged 51 in February 1972. He had a long history of skin disorders. During the latter part of 1971 he had constant trouble with ulceration and skin lesions on the left leg.

ii. The dressings of the leg were not done as frequently as they should have been. On two occasions Mr. Bartlett asked Mrs. Youell to do something about K's dressing. Mrs. Youell had to cut his sock, crepe bandage and swabs in order to get the dressing off. It is probable that he had been given a bath without renewing the dressing.

iii. In order to check whether the dressing was being done Mrs. Youell marked a swab which she applied to the leg on a Thursday night. The same swab was still on the leg when she checked on the following Sunday evening.

iv. Mrs. Youell told Mr. Large she had to dress K's leg. He told her that was a lie and that his nurses were very good.

v. Each ward had a treatment book in which any treatment required by a patient was entered. The procedure in Willows was that a student nurse would enter up the treatment required for each patient at the beginning of the week, obtaining the information from the medical records and, where appropriate, the entries of the previous week. There were spaces in the book for each nurse who carried out a treatment to initial the book to show that it had been done. Some did so, some did not.

vi. For each of the weeks from that commencing 8 January 1972 to that commencing 20 February 1972 the original entry of treatment for K was " Clean eyes apply Neosporin eye drop ". For each of these weeks Mr. Turkington added that a cream was to be applied to the leg. We are satisfied that the treatment for K's leg was not put in the treatment book until after Mrs. Youell had resigned and made her written complaints about the care of patients including the allegation that the dressings on K's leg had not been changed.

vii. Mr. Large and Mr. Turkington sometimes signed the treatment book after carrying out a dressing. On other occasions they did not do so. Although they were responsible for instructing student and pupil nurses how to carry out their work, neither of them gave any instructions as to how the treatment book was to be used.

viii. The recording of treatment that should be given was complicated by the fact that some of the treatment for patients who should have received daily baths was entered in the " bath book ". This book set out for each week the days upon which patients were due to have baths and contained columns for signature by staff to record that baths were in fact given. The system of keeping the book was as haphazard as that of the treatment book. Some staff signed the book after giving a bath, others did not. Neither Mr. Large nor Mr. Turkington gave any clear instructions as to what was required of the staff. There were undoubtedly times when baths could not be given on the due date because of shortage of staff, and there was one period of two or three months when the normal routine had to be abandoned because some of the baths were being changed and only one was available for use.

ix. The bath book contained the following entry for K "Apply calamine lotion to head. Betnovate ung to groin. Shave head PRN ". Between 2 January and 20 February 1972 K is initialled as having had a bath on four occasions, whereas he should have had one every day. We do not know how many baths he in fact received.

Comments

375. a. K did not receive proper care.
    b. Mr. Large and Mr. Turkington failed:
        i. to check that the dressings were being changed;
        ii. to see that the treatment and bath books were being properly kept.
    c. We consider at a later stage why this hopelessly haphazard and inefficient system was allowed to continue in Willows.

Patient Z

Facts found

376. i. Z was greatly troubled by boils on his back. In the ward report for the night of 13–14 February 1972 Mrs. Youell recorded that he was " very restless, kept getting out of bed to scratch his back on corner of door frame. He took the heads off the 4 boils on his back and kept scratching them. Boils cleaned and dressing applied but patient kept taking them off and was in quite a messy state. Patient was given a bath and painted with benzyl benzoate applied to all his body 12 midnight. He settled quickly and appears comfortable at time of report ".

    ii. As a result of Mrs. Youell's report Z was seen by Dr. Motashaw and Dr. Harfst on the afternoon of 14 February. Mr. Large recorded in the ward report that Gentian Violet was to be applied to the area of the boils.

    iii. When Mrs. Youell went on duty for the night of 14–15 February she found that there was no Gentian Violet.

Comment

377. This is another example of an unacceptably low standard of care.

Patient G

378. G was born on 6 March 1906 and died on 13 February 1972 as a result of severe internal injuries. No report of any kind of any incident which might account for the internal injuries was made until after his death. We therefore propose to report on the care of this patient in two sections. The first will deal with the care given to him in the villa. The second will consider the explanation put forward for the injuries.

Section 1

Facts found

379. i. G had been in Willows since November 1966. He was unable to give a clear account of himself or of time and place. He needed supervision in personal hygiene. He had a mental age of less than seven and suffered from a speech defect. He was very unsteady on his feet.

    ii. At 6.40 a.m. on 10 February G vomited a large amount of bile. Mrs. Youell had never seen anyone vomit so much bile before so she spoke to Mr. Macdonald who told her that Mr. Large was on his way to the villa. She entered in the ward report book that G had " vomited a large amount of bile 6.40 a.m. Apyrexial at time of report. Put to bed ". She spoke to Mr. Large about it when he arrived. Mr. Large gave G Horlicks for breakfast and he then got up. It was not uncommon for G to vomit. The following night Mrs. Youell noticed nothing unusual about G.

iii. On the night of 12–13 February Mrs. Copland was on duty. At 3.30 a.m. she found that G had vomited rather a large amount of " coffee grounds " vomit. That is dark brown vomit. She contacted Mr. Margan who told her to keep an eye on G and give him plenty of fluid. With difficulty she managed to persuade him to drink half a cup of water on two occasions.

iv. At 5.30 a.m. there was some projectile vomiting by G. Mrs. Copland noticed that there was a small bruise beginning to come up under his left eye and one on the bridge of his nose. Mrs. Copland again contacted Mr. Margan who came over to the villa on his bicycle. He looked at G and observed that the vomit was green in colour. He told Mrs. Copland to observe G for the rest of the night and they made him some tea of which he drank a little.

v. Mrs. Copland made a suitable entry in the ward report book and told Mr. Carim, who took over from her, what had occurred. After breakfast G again vomited " coffee grounds " and Dr. Benton was called to the villa and examined him at about 8.30 a.m. Dr. Benton found G looking sick. His pulse rate was about 96 and his blood pressure about 130/70. He did not appear to have a temperature. There was no evidence of tenderness or rigidity in the abdomen. In addition to the bruising observed by Mrs. Copland Dr. Benton noticed dried blood which appeared fresh in G's nostrils. She was unable to make a diagnosis and arranged for G to be transferred to the Gloucester Clinic. The transfer occurred at 10.30 a.m.

vi. At about midday Dr. Benton was called to the clinic and found that G " was in a state of extreme shock. He was very collapsed. It was impossible to feel his pulse or record his blood pressure. . . . His abdomen at this time was distended and somewhat rigid ". At 12.40 p.m. G produced a large quantity of vomit and died.

vii. Dr. Cameron carried out a post-mortem examination on 15 February. He found the following injuries:

a. External examination of the head showed an area of bruising in the middle of the lower forehead over the middle of the nose. It extended to the left side of the nose and above the left eye. There was also a small area of external bruising in the middle of the left forehead.

b. Internal examination of the head and neck revealed deep bruising over the prominence of both cheeks and in the middle of the forehead and over the left eye. There was bruising inside the upper lip and deep bruising over the left side of the voice box. There was slight bruising of the strap muscles covering the voice box on the left side of the neck. Dr. Cameron explained that by deep bruising he meant bruising of a deep nature which had not become

101

apparent externally before death. He said the delay in outward signs of deep bruising is common in elderly people, particularly those suffering from shock.

    c. External examination of the arms and legs showed bruising over the back of the left arm two inches below the elbow, lightly patterned abrasions over the outer side of the left elbow consistent with there having been clothing between skin and the object with which the elbow came into contact, and bruising on the inner side of the left knee.

    d. External examination of the abdomen revealed four distinct areas of bruising on the lower abdomen, three on the lower right and one on the lower left. They were linear in shape running across the abdomen.

    e. Internal examination of the abdomen revealed deep bruising of the abdominal wall particularly at the mid line and on either side of the navel. The mesentery was markedly swollen as a result of extensive bruising of the fatty tissue anchoring it to the back wall of the body. The mesentery lies two to three inches from the front of the body. The injuries to the abdomen and mesentery must have been inflicted from the front.

    f. There was external and quite severe deep bruising covering virtually the whole of the left testicle.

  viii. Dr. Cameron concluded that death was due to shock following severe bruising.

Comments on Section 1

380. a. Mr. Large should have asked a doctor to see G on the morning of 10 February. We consider that he tended to discount any report coming from Mrs. Youell. The vomiting on this occasion was not connected with G's death.

    b. Mr. Margan should have gone to Willows when informed that G had vomited "coffee grounds" at 3.30 a.m. on 13 February in order that he could decide for himself whether to call a doctor. It was Mrs. Copland's first night on duty in Willows and she did not know the patient. Vomit resembling coffee grounds often indicates that it contains blood.

    c. Mr. Margan should have called a doctor at 5.30 a.m.

Section 2

A. Steps taken by Mr. Large to find out what had happened to G

Facts found

381. i. Mr. Carim was on duty as charge nurse in Willows for the morning and afternoon shifts on 13 February. He recorded in the ward report book that bruising had been observed round G's left eye, that he had vomited "coffee grounds" after breakfast and that he had been transferred to the Gloucester Clinic where he had died at 12.40 p.m. He made a less detailed entry in the charge nurses' handover book.

ii. Mr. Large was on duty for both morning and afternoon shifts on 14 February. He read the report for the previous day but made no enquiries of anyone as to what had happened, even though he realised that G had vomited "coffee grounds" twice and had some bruising on his head. He was asked in relation to G's facial bruising, vomiting and death, "Although a number of patients were dying about this time, it was not a very usual occurrence, was it?" He replied " Well, it was not unusual because the only prognosis on that ward was death. They were geriatrics, and that was the only thing that could happen to them eventually ".

Comment

382. This last comment, coupled with the lack of interest in what had occurred, reveals an apathy and lack of concern which is entirely consistent with the unacceptably low standard of care in Willows.

B. The alleged explanation for G's injuries

383. Police enquiries started at once. On 15 February two ward orderlies, who had been on duty during Mr. Large's shift on the morning of 12 February and again during his shifts on 14 February, made statements about an incident which had occurred at the door leading from the day room to the toilet area at about 10 a.m. on 12 February. It was suggested to the Coroner's jury at Grays, Essex on 2 May 1972 that the evidence of these witnesses explained the injuries, and the jury returned a verdict of accidental death. We are satisfied that the occurrence at the door played no part in the injuries to the abdomen and testicle. We consider it unlikely that it caused all the remaining injuries. We propose to set out first the material evidence, and, secondly, our findings of fact.

Evidence

384. *Mr. Sharp* has now retired. We summarise his evidence thus:—

i. In February 1972 he was working as a ward orderly in Willows. He had held the job for about two years.

ii. At about 10.00 a.m. on 12 February 1972 the staff in the villa had their normal tea break at a table about halfway down the day room. The tea break lasted about twenty minutes, but all the staff were not at the table throughout that period. They sat looking in the general direction of the double doors leading out to the toilet area.

iii. There was a patient sitting in a wheelchair just inside the right hand of the two doors. He was often moved from this position as his chair prevented the right hand door from opening more than about 45°. The left hand door was normally bolted in a closed position.

iv. Mr. Sharp saw a young vigorous patient, W, move towards the doors during the tea break. If obstructed he would usually push the person or object out of the way.

v. As W reached the doors G was coming through the right hand door from the outside. It was partly open and G was entering the room sideways through the gap with his right shoulder coming into the room first. In order to get through between G and the left hand door W pushed him in the region of the back of the shoulder against the

103

right hand door which was thereby propelled violently against the wheelchair and rebounded against the upper part of the front of G's body throwing him backwards on to the floor of the day room. By this time W was out of the day room. Mr. Sharp at one time said that G landed on his face, but when he was referred to his statement to the police made on 15 February he said that he landed on his back and then rolled over on to his face. He was certain that G had never made contact with any part of the wheelchair.

    vi. G lay on the floor for a moment trying to get up before Mr. Sharp went to help him. He appeared " stunned—sort of knocked a little silly " for a few seconds and then seemed all right.

    vii. Mr. Sharp did not mention G's fall to anyone as there were other people who he assumed had seen what happened. He said Mr. Large was not in the day room at the time of G's fall. He did not know whether other members of the nursing staff were there.

385. *Mrs. Dawson*, a ward orderly, said :

    i. She heard Mr. Sharp say that W had pushed G over. She looked up and saw G with his back against the right hand door slowly sliding down the door. She was unable to see him when he reached the floor from where she was sitting.

    ii. She saw Mr. Sharp go to help G.

    iii. She believes that other members of the three nursing staff on duty were present at the time, but she could not say who.

386. *Mr. Charnier*, a student nurse, did not know if he was in the day room when the incident occurred.

387. *Mrs. Chatting*, a ward orderly, and *Mrs. Fynn*, a nursing assistant, saw nothing of the incident.

388. *Mr. Large* said he was called out of the day room during the tea break to answer the telephone. No-one told him of the incident.

389. *Dr. Cameron* said :

    i. the incident as described by Mr. Sharp could account for the injuries to the forehead, nose and area of the left eye, the cheek bones and the upper lip, but it could not account for the deep bruising of the voice box or the injuries to the abdomen or testicle.

    ii. the injuries to the abdomen would have required a " fairly severe degree of force ".

    iii. the abdominal injuries and those to the testicle could have been caused if G had come violently into contact with the edge of either an ordinary table or the table of a wheelchair.

    iv. G would have been winded and in pain immediately after the impact.

    v. all the injuries occurred at or about the same time. They could have occurred at any time up to three days before death.

390. We examined the door and were able to test how much rebound there was when it was thrown violently against a wheelchair. It was very slight.

391. We find:

  i. that a minor incident occurred in the doorway when W pushed past G. It is possible that the injuries to the forehead, face and lip were caused at this time.

  ii. that nothing occurred at that time which could account for the bruising of the abdomen and testicle. At no time in their evidence to us, or in their statements to the police, did Mr. Sharp or Mrs. Dawson suggest that G had come into contact with a table or wheelchair, or give a version of events consistent with that having occurred. Their statements to the police did not differ in any material particular from their evidence to us.

Comment

392. We are unable to decide how G sustained the injuries to his abdomen, testicle and voice box. We are satisfied that no further investigation will solve this mystery.

393. When we deal with the complaints by Mrs. Woods we will report on another incident involving G on 12 February. We are satisfied that he suffered no injury as a result of it.

Re-education of patients

394. Mrs. Youell told us, and we accept, that she spoke to Mr. Large about educating certain patients not to hit other patients. We also accept her evidence that nothing seemed to come from her requests.

395. The difficulties posed by Mrs. Youell's request are demonstrated by these facts and attitudes:

  i. Mr. Large said that there were at least twelve patients in Willows who had been violent to staff and patients during the twelve months before G's death.

  ii. Mrs. Youell explained how she dealt with this kind of behaviour. " Some of the patients look forward to outings very much, which they are getting a lot lately. . . . I knew that if these patients were told they could not go so-and-so if they continued to hit severely subnormal patients they would refrain, or try to refrain, from doing so, from the reaction I got from them. . . . The only weapon I had was a cup of tea in the morning. I could leave them without a cup of tea in the morning ".

  iii. Mr. Large and Mr. Turkington, however, took the view that privileges should never be withdrawn from patients. " If anybody did misbehave on the ward we spoke to them and tried to find out the cause of it before we even mentioned it to the doctor because we had to find out the grass roots ".

  iv. Miss Dooner, the Unit Nursing Officer, was aware of the problem caused by mixing old and young active patients, but did not appear to have any clear grasp of the numbers who were liable to push and hit others. She said she had discussed the problem of the mixed ages with Mr. Hubbard who had said that nothing could be done as this was a medical problem. She at no time discussed policy, as opposed to the treatment of individuals, with the doctors. No ward or case conferences took place in Willows until February 1972.

v. Occupational therapy only commenced in Willows early in 1972. A nurse comes to the ward for the purpose for six and a half hours daily from Monday to Friday and occupies twenty patients who were previously unoccupied.

vi. Student and pupil nurses formed at least half the nursing team. They have to move to another villa after about eight weeks under the rules laid down by the General Nursing Council and therefore never really get to know the patients.

Comment

396. There was an unacceptable lack of policy or guidance as to how the problems of misbehaviour by patients in Willows should be dealt with. This was common to the whole hospital. Many staff succeeded admirably. The less successful received no worthwhile assistance.

Mrs. Youell's Complaints of Administrative Deficiencies

397. We propose to deal with these very briefly. Mrs. Youell complained of the following matters:

i. *Mr. Large never went round the ward with her when she took over from him.* Mr. Large and some other witnesses said that he invariably went round. We find the truth lies somewhere between the two.

ii. *Mr. Large never read her " nursing notes " upon which she recorded information about patients which was not important enough for the ward report book.* We do not know if Mr. Large read the notes, but we are satisfied that he led Mrs. Youell to believe that he regarded them as a nuisance and of no value.

iii. *On her first night she was shocked to find that a number of patients kept buckets under their beds and urinated in them.* She managed to reduce the numbers to three by persuading the others to go to the toilet, but when she returned after a week's absence they had reverted to the use of buckets. When she complained to Mr. Margan he said the practice had been going on for years and that the patients were institutionalised. Mr. Margan told us that he disapproved of the use of the buckets but had done nothing to remove them. He did not like upsetting established customs. Mr. Macdonald said he did not know about the use of buckets until Mrs. Youell told him. He then asked her to remove all the buckets except two which belonged to patients who kept personal possessions in them. We find that Mrs. Youell's complaints were justified. The use of buckets for urination was a symptom of low care standards with no regard for individual dignity.

iv. *There was no PRN drug list.* Mrs. Youell told us that there had been such a list on other wards where she had worked and such lists saved her searching through the patients' records. We accept and endorse the evidence from other witnesses that PRN lists should not

106

be used: it is essential to work from the up-to-date medical records of each patient.

v. *No injection tray was laid out for her in the evening.* Mrs. Youell said that this was another practice followed on other wards and saved time. Mr. Large and other witnesses said that it was unnecessary and only saved two or three minutes. In our judgment an injection tray was not essential, but its absence in Willows was consistent with the low standards there.

vi. *The office cupboards were not labelled when she started work in December.* We find these complaints to be true.

vii. *Patients' records were in a muddle and the X-ray forms difficult to find.* We find these complaints to be true.

viii. *The names of dead patients were still on the bedding list and on the beds.* We find this complaint to be true.

ix. *The day staff sometimes left the villa unswept with pools of urine on the floor.* We find this complaint to be true.

x. *On occasions there was a flood in the toilets and they were dirty.* We find this complaint to be true. We accept Mr. Large's evidence that the pipes were too small and that the engineering staff had to clean them frequently.

General Conclusion as to Nursing Standards in Willows during December 1971 and January and February 1972

398. Care of patients during this period seldom exceeded the bare minimum and often fell below it.

How had this low standard of care been permitted to develop?

399. It is the responsibility of senior nursing staff and of medical staff to see that satisfactory standards of care are maintained in villas. We propose first to look at the attitude of Mr. Margan and Mr. Macdonald to Mrs. Youell's complaints, and then turn to the supervision by Miss Dooner and Mr. Hubbard.

400. *Mr. Margan* has worked at South Ockendon Hospital for sixteen years and has been a night charge nurse for about eight years. He had known Mrs. Youell since she started work at the hospital and had worked with her for three periods. He had a high regard for her as a nurse and found her a cheerful, uncomplaining person until January 1972. He said that she then became " very difficult to get on with. . . . My attitude towards this particular woman was that . . . I was anxious to have as little to do with her as possible ". He was asked if he could give a general picture of the sort of thing she complained about and replied " I cannot, really: just that she complained all the time. This is why I did not want to hang about there. I always wanted to see what was happening on the ward when she was on the ward, and then go. This complaining attitude was beginning to annoy me ". He thought her complaints were trivial and non-existent.

401. Later in his evidence he was reminded, and accepted, that he regarded her as a " very good and very conscientious nurse " and was asked:
Q. " So far as your dealings with her before were concerned, she had not been a complainer? " A. " I do not recall her being a complaining person.

I recall her being quite a happy kind of a woman, a lively person, a friendly person, quite a nice person to work with ".

Q. " Was it part of your duty to find out, if you could, from a nurse, particularly one with this background of very good, conscientious service, what it was that she really found unacceptable or difficult to work with on the ward ? " A. " Yes, I suppose it was, if you put it that way, but then again, remember, working in this atmosphere, meeting different nurses each night and so on, one does not always stop to consider ".

Q. " I am merely wanting to find out what the system was supposed to be. You accept that it was part of your duty to try and find out if you could what the trouble was ? " A. " If there was a complaint it was my duty to investigate it, but it was not necessarily my concern if a person was just having a grumbling nature. The woman may have had her private reasons for being like this. It was not up to me to probe into her domestic or private affairs or ask if she does not like me. She came to do her job and I came to do my job, and it was her job to do her job ".

402. A few questions later he agreed that one of Mrs. Youell's complaints had been that the patients were not getting a fair deal. The following questions and answers followed:—

Q. " But did you regard a complaint that patients were not getting a fair deal as a trivial matter ? " A. " The statement . . . that patients were not getting a fair deal is a statement which will indicate the kind of thing she was saying. I myself did not think the patients were not getting a fair deal. I thought they were as well treated on that ward as any other. . . . These complaints were unfounded. . . . I was quite satisfied with Willows Villa when I visited it at night ".

Q. " How long would you remain in the ward in the course of your routine visits ? " A. " It varied. . . . Anything from five minutes to half-an-hour depending on what was happening there ".

Q. "Are you meaning that you really disregarded [the complaints] and wrote them off as of no account because you on your very much shorter visits to the ward had not seen anything to support those comments by Mrs. Youell ? " A. " I saw nothing to indicate to me these were true. I could not see where the patients were deprived in any way. They seemed quite happy when they talked to me ".

Q. " So you pursued them no further with her ? " A. " That is true ".

403. *Mr. Macdonald* has been employed in nursing for 19 years and has been Night Superintendent of South Ockendon Hospital since August 1969. He said that from the end of January 1972 he had nightly complaints from Mrs. Youell, mainly about lack of co-operation from Mr. Large and pressure of work on her. He regarded the complaints as quite trivial and they were all settled to his satisfaction by him speaking to Mr. Large. He agreed that Mr. Large never disputed the validity of any complaint, but said that he would see that it did not happen again or some similar phrase. Mr. Macdonald said that Mrs. Youell had refused to put her complaints in writing and he had therefore not made any written report himself about them: he had, however, spoken to Miss Dooner, the Unit Nursing Officer.

404. We agree with Mrs. Youell that the attitude of Mr. Margan and Mr. Macdonald and others above her was " Don't look for trouble: take it easy ".

Mrs. Youell told us that Mr. Large informed her early in December that he had got rid of a nurse called Emambocus because he was always finding bruises and scratches on patients and making out accident reports. On looking at the appropriate records we established that Mr. Emambocus was on night duty in Willows from 31 December 1970 to 10 January 1971 and from 17 January to 31 January 1971. In that time he made out seven accident reports. Mr. Large said that he had no power to get rid of Mr. Emambocus himself, but he had spoken to his superiors about the accident reports made out by him. After the end of January 1971 Mr. Emambocus only did occasional night duty on Willows. We are satisfied that Mr. Large told Mrs. Youell that he had got rid of him, and that this assertion was probably correct.

405. *Miss Dooner* is a State Registered Nurse who served as an Assistant Matron at South Ockendon Hospital for 13 years. She attended a middle line management course at Oaklea College in 1969. She has been responsible for Willows Ward since December 1970 and was regraded as a Nursing Officer in February 1972. She is also the Nursing Officer for Hazels, Hawthorns and Hollies Villas. She is a shy person and had a very difficult job in Willows. We do not think she was able to exercise sufficient supervision in this villa, and we do not think that Mr. Large and Mr. Turkington paid much attention to her unless it suited them.

406. About 3 February Mr. Large asked her to move Mrs. Youell to another ward as there were personal difficulties between them. He never suggested that Mrs. Youell had been complaining of lack of co-operation or proper care of patients by him. Miss Dooner intended to speak to Mrs. Youell about the dispute, but was on leave from 4 to 14 February and did not have an opportunity to do so between her return and Mrs. Youell's resignation. She said that Mr. Macdonald had spoken to her once or twice about differences between Mrs. Youell and Mr. Large, but she had no clear recollection of what he had said.

407. *Mr. Hubbard* has been in the nursing profession for 34 years. He holds the following qualifications: State Registered Nurse, Registered Mental Nurse, Registered Nurse Mentally Subnormal, Registered Nurse Tutor. He came to South Ockendon Hospital in 1961 and was the Chief Male Nurse. In December 1971 he was appointed a Senior Nursing Officer with responsibility for 11 of the villas including Willows. He visited each villa at least once a fortnight.

408. Mr. Hubbard told us that about three or four years ago he had refused to issue instructions doing away with the treatment and bath books as recommended by a working party. He told us that it is the accepted practice that the bath book should be filled in with the dates on which patients are bathed, but there are no instructions about it. He left it entirely to the discretion of the Unit Nursing Officers to decide how often to check records. " They are totally responsible for their units ". He left it entirely to his Unit Nursing Officers' discretion as to how they should carry out their supervisory duties. " They have been placed under my control, and I have taken it for granted that they have been able and capable to carry out this sort of supervision. I have not issued any instructions at all ".

409. He was then asked:

Q. " So far as the treatment book is concerned what is the accepted practice as to that? We have heard Mr. Turkington give evidence saying that he really attached no importance to the signatures in the treatment books and gave no instructions to any student or pupil nurses in his ward about it . . .". A. "Again this is left to the discretion of the Nursing Officer and the charges of the ward. From my point of view I always like to see a signature ".

410. When Mr. Hubbard was asked whether he gave any indication to the officers under him about the kind of information he would like fed back to him " about nursing standards and so on " in villas, he said once again that he gave no such indication and left it entirely to their discretion.

411. It needs no words from us to indicate why the nursing service failed to detect or halt the declining standards in Willows Villa. Criticism from those below was resented and ignored wherever possible. There was a reluctance to give any subordinate any clear directions.

412. In making this criticism of the nursing supervision in Willows we are not denying that it is difficult to draw the line between nagging interference and unostentatious support and guidance. The qualities required are positive leadership and faith in one's own judgment. This will not be forthcoming if people without the necessary personal qualities are asked to do this important work. If they are lacking, the Salmon structure will create new and formidable problems. We recognise that its introduction poses acute problems as to how best to employ some people with many years of nursing experience who have not reached retiring age.

413. The conflict between villa autonomy and outside supervision was forcefully conveyed to us by part of the evidence of a young and energetic charge nurse, Mr. Bird. He is a State Registered Nurse and Registered Nurse Mentally Subnormal. He trained at South Ockendon Hospital from 1959 to 1962 and returned to South Ockendon Hospital as a charge nurse in 1969. He is branch secretary of Confederation of Health Service Employees.

414. He told us "As a charge nurse I am head of a household, therefore a person resistant to outside peering and prying eyes, as indeed is any person to interference from outside into the home. You may consider this to be an outdated idea, not in keeping with modern ideas of management. That is your prerogative. But it sums up my attitude to my work, and it is an attitude that has worked well and given proven results of its effectiveness ".

415. We asked him later in his evidence to explain his resistance to prying eyes. He said " I believe most sincerely that a person in charge of a caring team is the head of a household. I am the father of a large family myself, and if some neighbour comes to me with one of my children by the ear and says there is something wrong, I feel aggressive to the person who is the complainer. This is the reaction of a father. The reaction I am trying to convey to you about the charge nurse is that he reacts in that way ".

Q. " In the outside world at any rate, there are some good fathers, some bad fathers and a lot of pretty mediocre ones. I expect you have the same kind of situation with charge nurses. There are some good, there are some bad and there are some mediocre ?" A. " I agree ".

Q. " Supposing you have the mediocre or the bad charge nurse, the mediocre-to-bad, who is resistant to prying eyes from the outside on the kind of basis that you have been saying, how is that matter really dealt with? "

A. " I think you are asking me an unfair question. It strikes me that you are asking me to consider myself to be a different person than I am."

Q. " I am not, Mr. Bird. I am really asking your help on what I feel personally to be one of the antecedents to this Inquiry. How do you personally think, as a nurse with wide experience, this kind of situation should be dealt with? On the one hand you are—and I can understand the point of view precisely—saying ' if I am a charge nurse I should be left without prying eyes from outside to get on and do a really good job as I would do with my own family at home '. I can understand it completely, but what do you do with the fallibility of human nature when you have perhaps the rather poorer charge nurse who is not doing such a good job, not doing nearly as well as he could, who adopts the same attitude, ' Well I am the absolute father of this villa and nobody is to interfere? ' I hope you do not think it is unfair of me to ask you to express a view upon that dilemma which stems from your own assertion of the virtues of the resistance to prying eyes." A. " I understand now because you have expressed it differently. I think this is what the nursing officer is for. The nursing officer, or the assistant chief as he was before, should be aware that a person is behaving incorrectly, and if he is, his job is to counsel the charge nurse. If he requires reinforcement he should perhaps be taken out and given further training ".

Q. " The charge nurse might be resistant to the counselling, basing his resistance on what you say, ' Well I am the absolute authority here, I ought to be left to get on with it as a father with my own children '. Do you personally see this as a possible problem of attitude, that just as the good charge nurse might resent counselling based upon this particular way of thinking, so the poorer one might resist it for the same reason? " A. " I suggest to you that people are chosen to do a job, and when they are first appointed to a job they are carefully monitored and gradually the domination from above gets less and then the people who administer the place realise that a person is capable of making his own decisions. They will help the chap who is not showing signs of ability to do this. There is a lot to be said for this new idea of first and second class charge nurses on this basis. In some places they have deputy charge nurses. This is one of the arguments in favour of that ".

Medical supervision

416. Mr. Large said that he received comparatively few visits from Dr. Harfst and it was Dr. Motashaw who did most of the routine work. She had only started work in the hospital in June 1971. The visits of Dr. Harfst should have been recorded in the ward report book. He is there shown as having attended the villa between 1 December 1971 and 20 February 1972 on 13 December and 17 December, 7 January and 4 and 15 February. General medical care was on occasions below that which we would have hoped for and expected to find. Instead of lifting low nursing standards, the medical staff on occasions have accepted and adopted them.

The allegations of Mrs. Woods

417. *Mrs Woods* worked as a pupil nurse at South Ockendon Hospital from September 1971 to 8 September 1972. She resigned because of ill-health. In

February 1972 she was working in Willows Villa. We summarise her evidence thus:

i. On a Wednesday in the early part of February she saw Mr. Aboo Auchoybur, a pupil nurse, trip a patient, QQ, in the day room. Mr. Auchoybur thought it very funny. She made a note of the incident that evening at the end of her diary. We examined her diary and observed that she had used the end pages to record other occurrences.

ii. On another occasion early in February she saw Mr. Auchoybur trip up a patient, H, who is unsteady on his feet.

iii. On several occasions at the end of meals Mr. Auchoybur took a handkerchief out of the pocket of a patient, RR. He and Mrs. Anita Balah would then throw it backwards and forwards to each other. They appeared to regard it as very funny, but it infuriated RR. On one occasion Mr. Auchoybur hit RR on the head with a rag doll. RR retaliated by picking up a chair to hit Mr. Auchoybur. Mrs. Woods made a note of this incident on the bottom of her apron. We examined the apron and saw that she had used it for making other notes.

iv. On 12 February at about 6.00 p.m. she saw Mrs. Balah giving G a bath. She said it was not his usual day, but the routine in the bath book was not always followed. G was naked and approached the bath near the radiator very slowly. Mrs. Balah asked him to hurry up, but he could not come any more quickly. She put out her right arm and pulled him by the left wrist; she also put out her leg and put her foot behind one of his legs and tapped it on the back to make him move faster. Mrs. Woods asked if she could help and Mrs. Balah told her to leave him alone and not spoil him. G managed to get one leg slowly into the bath, but he then slipped and fell backwards into the bath hitting his back on the edge.

v. Incidents of the kind described in i, ii and iii above were regarded as a joke among the staff generally, including at least one charge nurse.

vi. She told Mrs. Youell about the earlier incidents. Mrs. Youell told her to speak to Mr. Turkington about them, but she did not do so, partly because she did not think he would believe her, and partly because she was afraid of losing her job.

vii. When she was seen by the police on 15 February in the course of their enquiries into the death of G she said nothing about these incidents, but said that she had information she was afraid to tell. The police asked if it would be easier for her if they came to her house. She agreed, and they went to her home on 17 February and took a second statement from her in which she referred to each of the above incidents and showed them her diary and apron which the police retained in their possession.

418. *Mr. Auchoybur* has been a pupil nurse since mid 1970. He denied that he had ever tripped any patient. He agreed that RR particularly liked to have a handkerchief, but denied that he had ever taken it from him. He said that G missed his normal bath on Friday, but denied that he was given one on the Saturday instead.

112

419. Mrs. Balah has been a nursing assistant since July 1970. She denied throwing RR's handkerchief about. She agreed that G had missed his bath on the Friday, but denied that he was given it on the Saturday.

Findings of fact

420. We accept Mrs. Wood's evidence as summarised above.

Comment

421. i. This is a further indication of a totally unacceptable standard of care in Willows. We doubt whether Mr. Auchoybur and Mrs. Balah realised how cruel their behaviour was. If the charge nurses had been doing their job properly it would not have occurred.
     ii. Mrs. Woods' fear of reporting such incidents was genuine. We encountered no witnesses of ill-treatment who did not share a similar fear. Mrs. Youell told us, and we accept, that she has been ostracised by many of the hospital staff, while others have told her that nothing will make them complain after seeing what has happened to her.

The present

422. We visited Willows on two occasions. We were glad to see that the enclosing of the verandahs had provided more space for activities and that occupation was now provided for many of the patients by staff from the Activities Centre, but the deployment of nursing resources that we saw on our visit did not encourage us to feel that all the problems had been dealt with adequately.

CHAPTER VII

OTHER VILLAS

423. South Ockendon Hospital has 22 wards, including two in the Gloucester Clinic. It was clearly not possible for us to investigate in depth the standard of care in all these wards. We were, however, able to form general impressions based on the letters we received from the relatives of present and former patients, and from voluntary helpers and staff, on the oral evidence given by some of them and on our own visits to the hospital. There was no formal programme for our visits and we walked round the hospital unaccompanied.

Letters

424. The bulk of the 253 letters we received came from relatives of patients or former patients. 21 were written by former members of staff, one by a member of the present staff. Replies came also from 3 former members of the Hospital Management Committee and from 3 organisations. There were 3 anonymous letters.

425. 70% of the letters praised the hospital and its staff. Most of them said that the staff did their best under difficult circumstances and some made suggestions on how things could be improved. One theme which occurred frequently in the letters was the kindness, and even love, which the nurses showed to the patients. One mother whose son has been a patient since 1958 wrote " I have never at any time seen anything but loving care and kindness given to all the patients . . . The staff care for each one of them with more patience and love than they would receive in many cases in their own homes ". Another mother whose daughter died recently after 11 years in the hospital wrote: " Wonderful people looked after her for me. They worried over her and tried their very best for her. . . . I used to visit (her) at odd times as well as normal visiting hours and always she was 100% cared for. . . . I loved my daughter very much and I admit I was scared to leave her 11 years ago because of talk of what happens in those places. I need not have been ". Another writer, whose aunt is in the hospital, said " We have only ever seen patience, understanding and *yes love* in dealing with the patients ". This lady gave oral evidence and, as she had visited her aunt regularly for more than 20 years, was able to describe the changes that had occurred during this period. She said that she had noticed an immense improvement since 1950 and that there had been marked improvement over the past three years, particularly as regards clothing, food and occupation. " She (her aunt) has far more to do now ". Apart from doing work outside the ward such as putting tops on washing up liquid bottles, she has also within the last 6 months been encouraged to make the beds: " She wheels her wheelchair round and makes the beds. They encourage her and she is paid for it . . . She likes us to take her books to colour and also most of the patients who can do them have puzzles to fit in ".

426. Another theme which appeared in several letters was the patients' pleasure in returning to the hospital after visiting home. For example:

" When he comes home for a change he always seems anxious to return ".
" My son has been at South Ockendon Hospital in temporary care for 3 weeks now and then, and he has been well looked after. Last time he did not want to come home ".

427. At least 40 writers commented that the hospital was understaffed. For example:

" On the many occasions that I made unannounced visits to South Ockendon Hospital I saw nothing but a very overworked nursing staff trying very hard and with seemingly endless patience, to cope with an impossible situation of very overcrowded wards and a severe shortage of staff and facilities. I have nothing but praise for the wonderful nursing staff . . . during the 7–8 years of my son's stay there. They have educated and trained him in a manner which to my way of thinking is beyond praise ".

" Children of this kind are heartbreaking to deal with, and the devotion of the staff operating in usually very understaffed conditions command nothing but my admiration ".

" The nurses and sisters were always cheerful in spite of the severe nursing shortage which is the reason for our only complaint—that (her daughter) spent too long in her cot and there was no time for exercise and therapy which she is getting now and which is obviously doing her a lot of good as is the extra love and attention at Little Highwood ".

" Our only complaint (if you can call it as such) is that we find the hospital is rather understaffed—and owing to same the inmates have a tendency of hurting one another. My daughter in particular has been scratched and even bitten in the past, also, sometimes we have noticed a lack of attention regarding her personal hygiene. This we cannot blame the staff for—for it must be quite a problem to attend to approximately 60 inmates—with just a sister and 2 nurses in attendance ".

428. About 50 letters made suggestions for improvement or criticised particular aspects of care. The main subjects mentioned were unsuitable clothing and the need for smaller groups and a more homely environment. Examples are:

" Clothing also needs more attention. If these handicapped people are to be accepted by the community their appearance must be made more acceptable. There is no room for lockers so clothing is all put together. This must cause the staff extra work sorting out sizes. For several weeks my son's trousers were so large round the waist he had to keep his hands in his pockets to hold them up. Then he came out with trousers about 6 inches too short . . . Women patients should not be sent out in short white socks. I realise this is easier to manage but it draws attention when they are outside the hospital and cannot be warm enough in winter ".

" Children were out walking . . . but wearing clothes that could only be described as ill-fitting and certainly owing nothing to fashion ".

" I have long been of the opinion that smaller groups of patients would help the staff in the practical application of care and to some extent prevent them being overwhelmed by their task, also giving greater opportunity to get to know their charges better ".

" Everything possible should be done to cast aside the ' institution ' and create a ' home '. In my daughter's villa I find the amenities and social provisions have greatly improved and a homelier atmosphere prevails. This is due to the forward-looking efforts of the staff, who are, however, dependent on the co-operation of the Hospital Management Board, who no doubt rely on Government grants for financial assistance. In the case of people like my daughter who have been used to the privacy of their own rooms, smaller units would have a beneficial effect. She is not an unfriendly girl but to be thrust day and night into company, crowded, perhaps aggressive, noisy and all strange cannot surely help any nervous disorder. Smaller units depend on more staff . . . Surely small units nearer each town would attract more auxiliary help which would release nurses for the bad cases which really need more attention ".

429. Pocket money or the absence of it, was mentioned in several letters and also the need to teach patients how to spend and how to save.

" My son has been in the hospital and has no idea of money and how to spend it. Perhaps there can be a way for these persons to try and learn about it, also we like to see them have a bit of pocket money as we take our son out every week and try to get him to shop a little for himself ".

" I feel a thrift book should be allowed to enable patients to save for anything special for themselves ".

" It would be nice if he had some money to spend when I get him every Sunday and when I bring him home for holidays. He likes to buy some things for himself ".

430. Several writers criticised the attention paid to physical illnesses and conditions, and several were worried about the mixing of different types of patients on the same ward. One complained of excessive drugging.

" There is sometimes less attention to the patients' wellbeing and comfort in relatively trivial aspects than one would wish. Minor medical conditions which appear fairly obvious have been unnoticed or untreated ".

" I myself attend to cutting of nails and treatment to his feet as he suffers with athlete's feet, but if it wasn't for my careful attention on many things I often wonder how he would fare ".

"At one stage his teeth were green near the gums. Some parents visiting regularly take a toothbrush etc and clean their children's teeth so it is done properly at least once a week . . . The hospital dentist informs me it is almost impossible to fill a mentally handicapped person's teeth and as hardly any of them can cope with false teeth many seemed destined to eat only soft foods from an early age. More attention should therefore be given to teeth hygiene ".

" When we brought her home she looked ill, hardly spoke and was obviously doped to the eyebrows. I had to keep her away from her Junior Training Centre for 2 weeks until the effects of the extra drugs wore off ".

" Each time I have my son . . . home he seems thinner and thinner and I worry a lot about him ".

" She certainly has put on a great deal of weight which is a great anxiety to me ".

431. A particularly interesting letter was one from a master of the Abbs Cross Technical High School which had been signed by two other masters also. The letter told us that pupils from the school started visiting in July 1967 and groups of pupils had been going, mainly in school term time, ever since, the main visiting

116

being on Wednesday evenings when normally about 25 pupils went and also occasionally at weekends. Six members of the school staff have also visited. The wards visited are Lindens, Laurels, Firs, Elms, Maples, Redmayes, Cedars, Hawthorns, and Larches; other wards have been visited occasionally. The age of the pupils varies from $14\frac{1}{2}$ to 18 and most are in the hospital for about two hours a week. The pupils go into the wards and chat to those amongst the patients with whom they are able to strike up a relationship. Those who are more self-assured go beyond this by helping patients in many ways. The comments of pupils and staff have been collected and were found to be almost wholly positive. " Many have been amazed at the tolerance and patience shown by the staff when dealing with patients, especially those who are anti-social or rather physical. . . . I cannot ever recall any child complaining that a member of the hospital staff had been deliberately or unwittingly cruel in dealing with a patient whilst the volunteers were there. The only comments on physical force I have heard have been where staff have been restraining rather aggressive patients. My experience is similar: I cannot recall having ever seen or heard a member of the hospital staff act in any other than a totally reasonable way. Having said this, there has been one constant vein of comparative criticism over the years. Many pupils have expressed surprise at the small number of staff on the villas at the times of our visits. There often appeared to be as few as 3 or 4 members of staff in a villa when we visit. The resultant lack of individual attention for some of the patients has concerned some of our visitors . . . I know that our voluntary helpers see a small part of the hospital for a tiny fraction of the time each week, but, given that limitation, I think we can offer virtually unstinted praise for what we have seen. . . . Perhaps a summary would be that it appears to us that the hospital staff contains many able, kind hearted people who make excellent relationships with the patients, but who seem to be operating in an inadequate system insofar as there seem to be too few staff and too many patients for the sort of personal help that many of the latter seem to need ".

Impressions gained from visits

432. We spent three whole days in visiting South Ockendon Hospital. Every villa was seen by at least two of us, and some villas were visited several times. We saw different aspects of the daily routine in one or other of the villas at all times of the day from early morning, before the night staff went off duty, until early evening when patients began to go to bed.

433. The standard of accommodation varies from very high to poor. At one extreme there are villas which have been upgraded by the provision of partitions to subdivide the dormitories and improved sanitary accommodation, and have been recently redecorated and completely refurnished. These villas, with their gay curtains, carpets, armchairs, modern beds and wardrobes or lockers for each patient are delightful. At the other extreme there are villas which have had only minimal improvements made to them and which are badly in need of redecoration and refurnishing; these have bare linoleum-covered floors, hard chairs and few and shabby armchairs. Their large dormitories have rows of iron beds much too close together.

434. Upgrading, if wrongly conceived, may produce its own problems. We were astonished to find that the two Laurels wards, created at some considerable expense by dividing a pre-war 2-storey villa, each provided a battery of W.Cs.

which were completely unscreened from the corridors along which all visitors must pass. There is an urgent need to remedy this affront to human dignity.

435. Generally the poorest accommodation is occupied by the most difficult patients, the severely subnormal and disturbed men and boys, and it is not easy to distinguish between cause and effect. There is a vicious circle of destructive behaviour, damaged furniture, dirty W.Cs., smell and a general lowering of standards. We found that the villas for women patients were usually brighter and more attractive than those for men and boys, though there were exceptions. Even the villa for disturbed women patients had a pleasant appearance, very different from that of Beech, the villa for disturbed men and boys which was built to the same design. Here again, cause and effect are intertwined. Severely subnormal women will often take a greater interest in, and be more willing to look after, such things as pretty carpets and counterpanes than will severely subnormal men.

436. Overcrowding remains a serious problem. The hospital as a whole provides, on average, at least 50 square feet bed space and 30 square feet day space for its patients. This is not the same as satisfying in each villa the minimum standard that hospital authorities were asked by the Department to achieve by December 1974, namely, providing in the wards at least 50 square feet of bed space and 30 square feet of day space for each patient. In several villas both the day and the night space available is below this minimum standard. Cypress is the only villa which satisfies the longer term objective of 70 square feet bed space and 48 square feet day space for each patient. Overcrowding is not only a matter of day and night space per patient in the villa. It is also affected by the type of patient and the amount of time spent by patients in the villa itself. More space is in our opinion needed in those villas where patients are unable to attend the Occupational Therapy Department or Activities Centre or to go to school. We found that some villas had managed to achieve a reasonable standard of care despite having less than the minimum space requirement. It was very clear that the dominating factor was the quality of the staff.

437. Unless staff are to accompany their patients to their various activities, it is necessary, when allocating staff to wards, to have regard to the situation at different times of the day and this obviously presents difficulties. It is a problem that has not always been successfully mastered at South Ockendon Hospital. For example, a pleasantly furnished villa for 55 subnormal and severely subnormal women which we visited at about 3.15 one afternoon had a staff nurse and an enrolled nurse on duty but all the patients were out. We had come straight from a villa for 37 severely subnormal and physically handicapped boys where there was only a student nurse in charge with another student, 2 pupils and 2 nursing assistants to assist him with the 15 children left in the villa. These children, unable to go out to school, appeared to be receiving no positive entertainment or training from a staff large in numbers but inadequate in competence. The general standard of care in this villa was one of the lowest we saw.

438. Another villa for about 40 subnormal and severely subnormal boys, which we visited earlier on the same afternoon presented a similar staffing picture of numbers without leadership, with the same depressing effect on the standard of care. Here a pupil nurse was in charge (in the temporary absence of the charge nurse) helped by a student and 2 nursing assistants. The pupil in charge was

uncertain how many patients there were in the villa: it transpired that there were 4 children and they were all running round aimlessly in the " bowl room " where the only member of staff present was preoccupied with sorting clothing. The opening of a cupboard revealed an appalling jumble of shoes with no name markings. From the replies we received to our questions it was clear that the staff had no idea to which child each shoe belonged.

439. It is only fair to say that both these children's villas had been mentioned by name in letters sent to us by parents praising the care given to their children at South Ockendon Hospital. We hope therefore that their unsatisfactory condition on the day of our visit was a temporary one.

440. The variation in the standards in the villas seemed to us to be typical of the good and bad features of the management of this hospital. The organisation is one which permits but does not insist on good standards. The high standard in a particular villa seems to depend on the personality and drive of a consultant or a charge nurse or some other individual on the medical or nursing staff. Where the standard is low and the ward staff are overwhelmed by their problems there is a lack of practical assistance and leadership from middle and top management. We heard often of the requirement on charge nurses to " act up " during absences of their Nursing Officers. In some wards we should have been glad to see a Nursing Officer " acting down " for a time.

Gloucester Clinic

441. The treatment centre in Gloucester Clinic has been referred to several times in earlier chapters. Its standard of care is high and it was universally praised.

Gloucester Drive

442. Earlier this year the unit known as Gloucester Drive was opened. It consists of a terrace of six single-storey houses, each containing three single bedrooms (attractively furnished and with full scope for personal possessions), a sitting room, kitchen and bathroom. Three high grade patients live in each* of these bungalows, doing most of their own cooking, washing and household chores. Here they are trained to prepare themselves for life outside the hospital by Mrs. Peggs, ward sister, and Mr. Bird, charge nurse, both of whom gave evidence to us. Mrs. Peggs explained that life in the ordinary wards had tended to take patients' usefulness away from them " because there are not the facilities in the ward to let them do their own cooking, and this type of thing ", so they need a great deal of training in basic household management and in everything they are going to need when living in the community. Evening classes are also arranged for the residents " where we teach them hobbies, because one of their main things is the lack of knowing what to do with their spare time ". The subjects include mending and making clothes, knitting, embroidery, washing and ironing and woodwork. There is a weekly meeting with the consultants, the psychologist and the social worker where the residents say what they want to say. There is also a residents' association, whose meetings are held on a Sunday afternoon, where the residents can voice all their complaints.

---

* Except one where only two patients reside, the third room being used as an office.

119

443. Apart from a few basic rules made by the consultant, all rules are made by the residents themselves.

444. The hospital is trying hard to get jobs for the residents and to arrange their admission into hostels or their return home. So far two have been discharged on trial leave.

445. We were very pleased to accept an invitation to tea at one of the bungalows and much enjoyed the cakes and sandwiches prepared by the residents.

446. The whole of this scheme seemed to us admirable in conception, and although it is too early to judge the effectiveness of its implementation, the management appear to have made a good start.

CHAPTER VIII

OCCUPATION AND RECREATION

447. A patient in South Ockendon Hospital, unless he is physically ill, is likely to be up by about 7.00 a.m.; if he wakes early and is restless he will get up much earlier. He will go to bed at some time between 5.00 and 10.00 p.m. How are these ten or more hours filled by people with little or no capacity for self-entertainment? A good deal of time is inevitably spent on the basic necessities of feeding or being fed, washing or being washed, and waiting for a turn for attention from busy staff. But there remain many long hours which, if unoccupied, allow passive patients to sink into apathy and hyperactive patients to erupt into violence and destruction.

448. In the early years of the National Health Service the many able-bodied high grade patients worked hard in the wards, the kitchens, the laundry or outside in the gardens or on farms. Others exerted themselves in hospital workshops making and repairing the various items of furniture and clothing needed by the hospital.

449. In South Ockendon Hospital the only remaining trace of these thriving workshops is the upholstery department in the Industrial Therapy building. Few of the patients in South Ockendon today are capable of skilled work.

450. This change in the patient population is the outcome of the successful drive to rehabilitate patients capable of returning to the community, combined with changes in medical knowledge and practice which have resulted in severely handicapped babies surviving, when previously they would have died, and in handicapped people living into old age when previously their life span was shorter.

451. The result is that in the Occupational Therapy Department, in the Industrial Therapy Department and Activities Centre and in the wards it has been necessary to find new forms of work and recreation suitable for the capacities of the patients. In all these places shortage of staff prevents development to the extent needed.

Occupational Therapy Department

452. The Occupational Therapy Department is in a modern purpose built building. The Head Occupational Therapist, Miss Gibberd, has 18 part-time assistants, none of whom is a qualified occupational therapist. 113 patients attend the Occupational Therapy Department. They do painting, music and movement and mime and a little drama; they also do needlework, woodwork, papier mache, knitting and some domestic science and cooking. Miss Gibberd told us that since more seriously subnormal patients had been attending the department, she had had to change the occupations to suit their abilities. There was no space to take more patients and she felt that her staff were all needed

in the department and could not be spared to take occupational therapy classes in the wards. With limited space and staff she could not deal with more than a few patients with behaviour problems.

Industrial Therapy Department and Activities Cntre

453. Many activities similar to those in the Occupational Therapy Department are also carried on in another, older building which functions separately under Mr. G. F. Wood, who has been Officer in Charge of Patients' Work and Activities since May 1972. He is a Grade 7 Nursing Officer responsible to the Principal Nursing Officer. In the Industrial Therapy Section of this building 125 patients are engaged mainly in light assembly and packaging work. In the Activities Section, a further 114 more severely handicapped patients are occupied with play, music, painting, drawing, construction toys and other simple diversions. Many of the patients are overactive, and for their benefit, in particular, the day's programme also includes long walks with visits to the adventure playground. 30 more patients spend part of each day either in the Activities Centre or in the Occupational Therapy Department; these include small groups of disturbed patients from Cypress, Beech and Poplars wards, who come for only short periods.

454. Shortage of space limits the number of patients who can attend the Industrial Therapy Department and Activities Centre but Mr. Wood has established ward activity groups—so far in only three wards—by allocating nursing staff to these wards for the specific purpose of occupying patients on the ward. At present 51 patients are occupied from 9.00 a.m. until 5.00 p.m. in these groups. Mr. Wood explained that when ward staff were short recreational activities were the first to be set aside. " The idea of putting a nurse specifically on these wards to do these activities was so that these things could go on irrespective of the demands made on other staff ". Mr. Wood, with a staff of 23, including 3 nurses and 3 to 4 nurse learners, covers Industrial Therapy, the Activities Centre and the three ward activity groups, and estimated that he needed a staff of about 40 to cope adequately with the existing patients in the existing premises; it would then be possible to reduce the size of the groups and give more individual attention to the patients.

Other Occupations

455. 106 other patients are occupied in various ways. Five of them are gainfully employed outside the hospital: 55 are employed in domestic work in the hospital, 34 in the departments as, for example, kitchen porters, and 12 in the farm and gardens.

Education

456. There are 86 children aged from 5–19 on the roll of the hospital school run by the local education authority. The Headmistress, Miss Hutterer, has a deputy, Mrs. O'Shea, and 12 teachers. There are also six attendants to assist the teachers. The aim is to run the school as a normal school with defined periods for painting, habit training, hygiene and physical education, and with reading and writing for the few able to absorb these subjects. The children are also taken on excursions to visit such places as railway stations, airports and restaurants.

457. Miss Hutterer said that there were only about 15 children not attending the school and some of them were so severely multiply-handicapped that they could not get into the school. She had not been able to do much about reassessing rejected children and relied on the nursing staff to let her know if a child had become ready for schooling. New patients in the hospital were assessed by medical staff and were admitted to the school when next a vacancy occurred at the beginning of a term.

458. During school holidays nursing staff care for the children, the school premises being left open for their use. Mrs. Briggs said that the children were sent to holiday school when a nurse could be spared: that two members of the school staff came back by arrangement with the hospital: and in summer students were taken on to help.

459. 21 patients attend the Adult Training Centre, temporarily housed in the Activities Centre and staffed by teachers from Thurrock Technical College.

In the Wards

460. Some 230 patients have no occupation other than that which can be supplied by the hard-pressed ward staff. It was only too clear, on our visits to the hospital, that much of the time of these patients was empty of interest and stimulation. Toys and occupational equipment have been in unjustifiably short supply until about two years ago. Almost all that were bought came from money raised by the League of Friends. The money spent by the hospital on such equipment for the school and the rest of the hospital is set out below:

Year	School	Rest of Hospital	Total
1966/67	£341	—	£341
1967/68	£307	£82	£389
1968/69	£644	£41	£685
1969/70	£699	£12	£711
1970/71	£155	—	£155
1971/72	£545	£57	£602

The allocation for 1972/73 has been raised to £2000.

461. We accept the evidence that requests for more equipment were on some occasions turned down because of shortage of money. Mr. Whiting explained the dilemma of the Hospital Management Committee " It is all a question of priorities is it not? Do you paint the window frames to stop the glass falling out or do you provide play equipment? And this is the sort of problem which the Management Committee has been up against all the time I have been associated with it. The question of engineering and general building and maintenance is really the most pressing problem which the Management Committee has been engaged in all the time. . . . The Friends of South Ockendon decided to provide some incinerators to be placed on the female wards. In actual fact, we had to say to them ' We are sorry, but we simply cannot have them because we have not got enough money to install them '. Now that is a pretty drastic sort of a situation, and one then says, which is the more important thing? Is the installation of an incinerator on a ward more important than play equipment? You tell me the answer. I do not know. . . . The Friends of South Ockendon had X

123

thousand pounds, a very large sum of money, to provide a hydro therapy pool, and the Management Committee has to refuse to accept it because of the revenue consequences of its installation. This is a crazy situation, but it is not unique, you know ".

462. Mr. Whiting explained that the extra allocation for 1972/73 was possible because " we have had a number of supplementary sums of money thrown into our lap ".

463. We sympathise with the Management Committee in their dilemma, but we have no doubt that they have got their priorities wrong. More money should have been spent on play equipment even if maintenance of the buildings had suffered a little. We explain in a later section of this report why in our view the Hospital Management Committee got their priorities wrong.

464. There is now a toy bank from which wards can obtain play materials.

Recreation

465. Dr. Yorke-Moore, who has worked in seven hospitals, told us that South Ockendon Hospital had a long tradition in emphasising the value of recreation and that it compared very favourably with any other similar department he had known elsewhere.

466. The officer now in charge of patients' recreation is Mr. W. Davies, a Nursing Officer, with the assistance of a staff of six. For accommodation he had the use of the main hall and the annexe.

467. Mr. Davies described to us the extent of arrangements made for recreation, mainly in the evenings. The various clubs include a twice weekly mixed junior club which has organised team games, dancing, swimming and the trampoline; a weekly club for elderly semi-ambulant and non-ambulant men and women patients of both severely subnormal and subnormal grade, who are entertained with the playing of records and table games such as dominoes, ludo and cards: and a weekly club for severely subnormal men and women who have dancing, singing and organised games. There is also a voluntary youth club, run by a committee formed by various youth clubs in the area, which meets once a week when a dozen or so people from the youth clubs help with disco dances, bingo, table tennis, snooker, table games, painting and knitting.

468. For those severely subnormal or disturbed patients who cannot take part in the other clubs, activities are arranged on two evenings in the week by the Activities Officer in the Activity Centre: these patients play ball games, listen to records and have an occasional film show.

469. Cinema shows are held twice, or, in winter, three times a week, and in winter shows are also provided on the wards for patients who are unable to go out.

470. There are outings to places of interest, to seaside resorts, to concerts given by various schools, to pantomimes etc. Various organisations also visit the hospital to give concerts. Cricket, table tennis, snooker and darts are played in competition with other hospitals.

471. Mr. Davies said his greatest need was a big covered area for games and other boisterous activities in winter time, and his greatest problem was the finding of suitable staff who were prepared to work late in the evenings and to participate in the patients' activities. He had never been refused an increase in establishment; as suitable people came along, he was able to take them on. He habitually went out of the hospital to youth clubs and other organisations in order to awaken their interest, and he agreed that in this respect there was no rigid dividing line between his work and that of the Organiser of Voluntary Services. He also had good contact with the League of Hospital Friends.

Voluntary Services

472. The Group Organiser of Voluntary Services is Mr. G. L. Thomas. He has been instrumental in increasing the number of volunteers and has been particularly successful in obtaining the services of a large number of young people. Members of voluntary organisations and pupils of schools visit the hospital to give personal services to patients such as reading to them, writing letters for them, playing games and taking them for walks. Voluntary helpers organise outings and raise money for amenities. They have given their labour on the construction of the adventure playground and have made gifts of the necessary material and equipment. Altogether about 150 to 170 volunteers pass through the hospital each week doing various jobs, and this contact with the outside world is of immense benefit to the hospital and its patients.

473. There is an active League of Hospital Friends whose chairman, Mr. F. J. Pryor, gave evidence to us. The Friends with a membership of 250, of whom 30 or 40 are active, raise about £3,000 a year by raffles, a bazaar, selling Christmas cards and so on. They have pioneered the introduction of various pieces of new hospital equipment to see whether they would prove worthwhile. These include helmets for epileptic patients which have since been adopted by the hospital. The Friends also supplied spin-dryers to some villas at the request of the nursing staff who had volunteered to hand-wash woollen items. All unvisited patients are provided with birthday and Christmas presents.

474. Mr. Pryor said that relations with the hospital staff at all levels were good and he spoke highly of the standard of care that the nursing staff displayed to the patients. (His own daughter had been a patient from 1956 until her death in 1972.)

475. We heard from others of the help given, with advice or gifts, by particular voluntary organisations such as the local Society for Mentally Handicapped Children, the National Association for Mental Health, the Spastics Society and the Variety Club of Great Britain.

Initiatives at Ward Level

476. We heard from several sources of the independent progressive work done by ward staff over the last three or four years. A number of charge nurses have on their own initiative, and with the support of their Nursing Officers, developed schemes for their own villas such as an Open Day for parents and relatives, the formation of parents associations for individual wards, ward parties, ward outings, even a ward percussion band. Some had tried different methods of arranging the wards so as to enable the patients to be looked after

in smaller groups. Some had concentrated on habit training to reduce incontinence or on diversions to reduce disturbance. Others had made particular efforts to create a more home like appearance in the villa. One ward for disturbed women patients introduced a scheme for staff to take meals with the patients which proved of considerable benefit to the patients. We ourselves were very pleased to accept an invitation to have lunch on this ward, and we saw for ourselves how successful the arrangement was. Several of the charge nurses came to give evidence to us about what they had been doing, and we were impressed with their enthusiasm and their obvious pride and pleasure in what they had been able to achieve.

477. From Nursing Officers, we heard of the many occasions on which ward staff, both nursing and domestic, had given their off duty time to take patients on outings, to shop for them, to alter their dresses, make cakes for parties and in many other ways.

Comment

478. The present accommodation available for occupational and industrial therapy is inadequate. We are glad that it is to be extended. The planning and positioning of the new accommodation will need careful thought.

479. At present there are about 230 patients who do not leave the villas for any form of occupation. There are nurses working under Mr. Wood who bring activity and occupational therapy into three villas. The number of these workers needs to be substantially increased.

480. The allocation of human and material resources is unnecessarily complicated by the fact that the work of Mr. Wood (The Activities Officer) and Miss Gibberd (the Occupational Therapist) overlap. Much of the activity in the Activities Centre is indistinguishable from that in the Occupational Therapy building. Mr. Wood is responsible to the Chief Nursing Officer. Miss Gibberd regards herself as responsible to Dr. Dutton. We found that Mr. Wood's department was more outward looking and related more to the general life of the hospital than Miss Gibberd's department. We sensed that part of the problem is that Miss Gibberd feels that people without her specialised training who are not working under her immediate supervision cannot really understand her work. These barriers must be broken down. We suggest a framework within which this can be achieved later in this report. We emphasise at this stage that anyone who is unable, either through wish or temperament, to work as part of a team must be removed.

481. There is a great need for an indoor play centre where vigorous games can be played throughout the year. The use of drugs will fall if overactive patients are able to enjoy letting off their surplus physical energy.

482. Subject to the comments above we were greatly impressed by the imagination, enthusiasm and hard work displayed in these departments and organisations. Much of this activity could and should have started at an earlier date.

CHAPTER IX

GENERAL MATTERS

Management

483. Management is an essential part of the care of patients. If the function of management is regarded too narrowly the standard of care is likely to be unnecessarily low. What ought the aims of management to be at South Ockendon Hospital? In order to answer this question we must first look at the statutory duties as explained by Ministerial and Departmental Memoranda.

The Minister of Health (now the Secretary of State for Social Services)

484. a. Section 1 of the National Health Service Act 1946 provides " it shall be the duty of the Minister of Health—to promote the establishment in England and Wales* of a comprehensive health service designed to secure improvement in the physical and mental health of the people of England and Wales* and the prevention, diagnosis and treatment of illness, and for that purpose to provide or secure the effective provision of services in accordance with " the provisions of the Act.

b. Section 3(1) of the same Act states that " it shall be the duty of the Minister to provide throughout England and Wales* to such extent as he considers necessary to meet all reasonable requirements " hospital accommodation together with the medical, nursing and other services required at or for the purposes of such hospitals.

The Regional Hospital Board

485. a. Section 12(1) of the same Act states " Subject to the exercise of functions by Hospital Management Committees in accordance with the next following subsection, it shall be the duty of a Regional Hospital Board, subject to and in accordance with regulations and such directions as may be given by the Minister, generally to administer on behalf of the Minister the hospital and specialist services provided in their area, and in particular " to appoint the necessary officers, to maintain buildings and acquire and maintain equipment and furniture.

b. Regulations were made by the Minister which were described in R.H.B. (48)2 as having been " designed to confer on Regional Hospital Boards, acting as the Minister's agents, the powers necessary to enable them to guide and control the planning, conduct and development of services in their area ".

c. By Regulation 3 of the National Health Service (Functions of Regional Hospital Boards etc) Regulations 1969 the Secretary of State decided "A Regional Hospital Board shall, subject to and in accordance with these regulations and any directions which may be

---

*The Transfer of Function (Wales) Order 1969 transferred responsibility for provision of these services in Wales to the Secretary of State for Wales.

given by the Secretary of State, subject to the exercise of functions by Hospital Management Committees . . . administer on behalf of the Secretary of State the hospital and specialist services in their area ".

The Hospital Management Committee

486. a. Section 12(2) of the 1946 Act provides " It shall be the duty of the Hospital Management Committee of any hospital or group of hospitals, subject to and in accordance with regulations and such directions, as may be given by the Minister or the Regional Hospital Board, to control and manage that hospital or group of hospitals on behalf of the Board, and for that purpose to exercise on behalf of the Board such of the functions of the Board relating to that hospital or group of hospitals as may be prescribed ".

b. The 1948 regulations were described by R.H.B. (48)2 as conferring on Management Committees the " powers necessary to enable them to carry out the duty laid on them by section 12(2) of the Act to control and manage on behalf of the Regional Board the hospital or group of hospitals which they administer. The scope of the services to be provided at or in connection with the different hospitals will be determined by the policy of the Regional Board and the Minister; the task of the Management Committee will be to secure their efficient maintenance and administration . . . ".

c. Part of Regulation 5 of the 1969 Regulations provided " The Hospital Management Committee of any hospital or group of hospitals shall, subject to and in accordance with any directions which may be given by the Regional Hospital Board concerned or by the Secretary of State, control and manage the Hospital or group of hospitals and the services provided in connection therewith on behalf of the Board . . . ".

487. The duty cast upon the Minister was clearly expressed and unequivocal in its demands. It cannot be performed without adequate money, and nobody can doubt that the money allocated by Parliament has been inadequate.

488. The duty cast upon the Regional Hospitals Boards and Hospital Management Committees was not so clearly expressed. Nevertheless there should in our view have been no doubt that the duties laid on the Hospital Management Committees as agents for the Boards included that of ensuring that patients were properly cared for in the light of contemporary knowledge within the framework of any policy laid down by the Department or the Board. Neither should there have been any doubt that one of the duties of the Board was to ensure that their agents, the Hospital Management Committees, were carrying out their duty satisfactorily.

489. These duties could not be performed unless the Board and the Management Committee took steps to find out how the patients were cared for and gave any necessary directions to eliminate or reduce any defects they discovered. Boards do not appear to have understood this until the memorandum H.M. (69)59 issued in July 1969. The South Ockendon Group Hospital Management Committee in our view took a very restricted view of its duty.

The Regional Hospital Board

490. We have already said that the Board should have laid down a policy for Cypress Villa and taken steps to see whether it was functioning satisfactorily. (See paragraph 180.) Professor Ramsay seems to have thought that to do either would involve an unjustifiable and unacceptable encroachment on the clinical autonomy of the consultant. (See paragraphs 212–215.)

491. We have also said that the Board should have realised the dangers of overcrowding and understaffing at the hospital earlier than it did (see paragraph 142), and that in deciding what cuts to make in its 1962 10-year programme it took too sanguine a view of the number of hostel places that would be provided by local authorities. (See paragraph 32). The Board was wrong to appoint Mr. Nichols as Chairman of the Hospital Management Committee in 1969. (See paragraph 522). It failed to see that a sensible workable multi-disciplinary structure was in operation at the hospital after Dr. Dutton ceased to be Physician Superintendent in 1972. (See paragraphs 506 to 507).

The Hospital Management Committee

492. The names of the Hospital Management Committee are set out in Appendix 8. We heard evidence from the Chairman and Vice-Chairman and received written evidence from 8 other members. We met a number of them informally at lunch at the hospital on 31 July.

493. We have no doubt that they have at all times been a very hard working committee, but the many hours of work they have spent, both in Committee and in visiting, have in considerable part been misdirected.

494. In the first place they have taken a very restricted view of their duty towards the patients. We have already set out the Chairman's views in paragraphs 218–219. We have no reason to think that these were not a fair reflection of the views of the Committee as a whole. They wrongly, in our opinion, regarded the way of life in each villa as lying within the clinical autonomy of the consultants. Moreover they considered that the control and correction of the consultants must come from the Board who appointed them. Their insistence that they were mere laymen created an unreal mental barrier between themselves and the consultants, and tended to invest the consultants with an infallibility which few, if any, people in any walk of life possess. All these views unduly hampered their essential enquiring function. Many questions that should have been asked were not asked. Answers that should not have been accepted were too readily accepted. All people charged with the management of a hospital, whether laymen or professional, must have faith in their own judgment and in the evidence of their own eyes. If they feel that something is wrong they must ask questions until they are really satisfied. If they are not satisfied they must take appropriate action.

495. In his closing written submission to us Counsel on behalf of the Management Committee said " To put it simply the Hospital Management Committee has concerned itself with the physical needs and requirements of the patients leaving the professional matters of medical treatment and care to those qualified to give it. From a detailed examination of the minutes it can be seen that the only monitoring of the professional duties of the nurses and medical staff is by the examination in detail of any complaints that are made to the Hospital Management Committee from whatever source ". This restricted view of their function

really made the Management Committee little more than the supplier of " hotel services " in an " hotel " whose policy and management was left in the hands of the consultants.

496. He continued with an understatement. " This method of testing the standard of care being given to patients has been likened to a barometer or perhaps a thermometer, but such occasional temperature readings and the frequency of them is not necessarily a satisfactory guide as to the standard of nursing or medical care that is being given to patients ".

497. This concentration by the Management Committee on the physical conditions and their leaving of the way of life to the professionals was in our opinion responsible for their failure to spend sufficient on educational toys and equipment. (See paragraphs 460–461.) Unless the Management Committee concerned itself with the way of life they would not understand the importance of there being sufficient means of occupation and the extent to which occupation could affect patients' behaviour.

498. By leaving matters of policy largely in the hands of the consultants the Hospital Management Committee created a situation in which they concentrated on matters of detail which should have been dealt with by their officers. As a result of this limited role in which all at the hospital saw the Hospital Management Committee they were not given sufficient information presented in such a manner as to require decisions on matters of policy.

499. The ineffectiveness of the Management Committee and their reluctance to face up to important matters of principle and policy, instead of concerning themselves with a mass of detail, can be demonstrated by their attitude to the Hospital Advisory Service Report, the subcommittee structure, and representations which were received from a number of the charge nurses. We look at each of these in turn.

The Hospital Advisory Service Report

500. The Management Committee referred this Report to a small Subcommittee whose report was, as subsequently minuted, prepared rather hurriedly. We set out parts of the Hospital Advisory Service Report with the Subcommittee's comments.

501. *H.A.S. Paragraph 7.8* (last sentence). " There are also differences of opinion between medical and nursing staff and other inter-departmental disagreements which inevitably affect the overall therapeutic purpose of the hospital ".

502. *Subcommittee comment.* " The last sentence of the paragraph may be true in part but it is felt that it does not extend throughout the hospital. The comment does not identify clearly where the problem lies and the Hospital Management Committee feels that solutions can only be effected if generalised statements are made more specific ".

503. In our view this was an abdication of responsibility. Steps should have been taken to find out where the inter-departmental disagreements lay. The position of the Occupational Therapy Department should have been considered for a start.

504. *H.A.S. paragraph 11.3.* " The Physician Superintendent has an administrative responsibility for all units of the Group. This is onerous, demanding and time-consuming work. A Medical Advisory Committee is in existence and more recently a Division of Psychiatry has been established. There are therefore 3 systems of ' medical administration ' in being, and the functions of each in relation to the hospital and in relation to the Hospital Management Committee seem somewhat unclear ".

505. *Subcommittee comment.* " This paragraph may be misleading. In practice the Chairman of the Division of Psychiatry and the Physician Superintendent are the same person and this does not create problems ".

506. In fact the medical committee structure cried out for reorganisation. The function of the various committees and their relationship to each other was totally unclear. Early in 1969 following the publication of the first Cogwheel report the Medical Advisory Committee decided that a Psychiatric Division should be formed consisting of all the psychiatric staff in the Group. They decided subject to approval by the Board, that Dr. Dutton should be Chairman of that Division and also Chairman of a non-existent Medical Executive Committee. The Division would carry out the functions set out in paragraph 58 of the Cogwheel report and also that of the non-existent Medical Executive Committee as set out in paragraph 63 of the Cogwheel report. Thereafter the Medical Advisory Committee and the Psychiatric Division met together at the same time. No effort was made to distinguish between their functions or consider whether there was a need to retain both committees. We do not understand how the Management Committee approved such a structure. Still less do we understand how the Subcommittee could so lightly brush aside the Hospital Advisory Service comments upon it.

507. Later in 1971 the Medical Advisory Committee was abolished and the Medical Executive Committee of which Dr. Dutton was the Chairman and sole member was reinforced by all the Consultant Psychiatrists in the group. The Medical Executive Committee and the Psychiatric Division continued to meet together. In a letter to Dr. Ramsay dated 28 February 1972 the Group Secretary explained the position thus, " The Psychiatric Division and Medical Executive Committees are extensively coterminous and in practice usually meet synchronously ".

508. *H.A.S. Paragraph 29.1.* " It is obvious that this hospital has been labouring under very great difficulties for a long time. The combination of overcrowding, staff shortages and inadequate provisions for the occupation and training of patients give rise to a grave and undeniably dangerous situation. I consider that, while conditions remain as they are, the patients at this hospital remain at risk. There is a limit to the amount of stress which staff on high dependency wards can endure over a prolonged period. Moreover, there is no doubt that patients admitted to some areas within the hospital in the prevailing circumstances could only deteriorate ".

509. *Subcommittee comment.* " The Hospital Management Committee feels that if there is a ' grave and undeniably dangerous situation ' the present 1 in 4 admission policy should be re-examined. This paragraph expressed unequivocally the Hospital Advisory Service view of the situation at South Ockendon Hospital and is possibly the most important paragraph of the report ".

510. The word " if " is significant. There was, so far as we could ascertain, no finding by the Subcommittee or subsequent consideration by the Management Committee as to the validity of the comments in this important paragraph.

511. We asked Mr. Nichols " Did you ever come to the view that overcrowding and understaffing created a situation of danger for the patients? ". A. " I dare not say danger because we had a staff of doctors and nurses who would see to it that patients were never in danger as such. The hazards were always there because of lack of space . . . ".

Q. " Did you ever feel that, not through any lack of willingness on the part of the staff but because of shortage of staff and overcrowding, the care of patients had reached an unacceptably low level at any time? " A. " I could never accept that it was at a very low level. I reiterate we had a dedicated staff, and they did their best under the circumstances. I visited these hospitals, all of them within the Group, and in particular South Ockendon. Overcrowding was manifest, shortage of staff was there, but whatever loving care could be given was given, as you will know with possibly one or two exceptions. The best was given at all times within the resources available ". . . .

Q. " Mr. Nichols would you just take . . . the Hospital Advisory Service Report? It is . . . paragraph 29.1 ". A. " Yes, I am looking at that. I accept that, but do you want my frank answer to this, on this ' undeniably dangerous situation '? "

Q. " I was asking you to look at it . . . because I think you were saying that you could not accept that there was ever a dangerous situation or patients at risk, because of the dedication of the staff? " A. " Yes ".

Q. " When you received this report, did you as a Management Committee make up your minds whether that assessment of the position at the hospital was in your view a valid one or not? " A. " Well, you see, I have never accepted that ' dangerous ' was correct, because if there is a truly dangerous situation no responsible person would allow that to continue; you would probably close up the wards. It was a difficult and a serious and a grave situation, but I cannot accept that it was dangerous in the full sense of the word ".

512. Subsequent questions and answers failed to clarify further the views of the Subcommittee or Management Committee. In our view the dedication of the staff was being used as a mental shield against reality. However dedicated the staff might be it was probable that one or more would pass the limit of stress which they could endure. If that occurred patients were at risk and a situation of danger created. Quite apart from the stresses which some members of the staff would not be able to endure there was the danger to patients created by violence amongst themselves.

513. The report of the Subcommittee was laid before the Management Committee on 28 May 1971. It was minuted " It was agreed that as there had been insufficient time to consider the findings of the Subcommittee that members contact the Group Secretary indicating to him any further observations that needed to be incorporated so that all the views could be communicated in due course to the Regional Hospital Board ".

514. No members did communicate views to the Secretary and the Management Committee considered the report no further. It was left to the Regional Hospital Board.

The Subcommittee structure

515. There were four Subcommittees. 1, The Finance and General Purposes. 2, Land and Works. 3, Establishment. 4, Patients and Welfare. These and the Management Committee each met once a month except during August. In addition there were infrequent and irregular meetings of a Nursing Advisory and Education Committee and the Chairmen of Subcommittees.

516. We have read all the minutes between 1 January 1968 and August 1972. They show a concentration on matters of detail which should have been delegated to the Group Professional Executive Team consisting of the Physician Superintendent (latterly the Chairman of the Medical Executive Committee), the Group Secretary, the Chief Nursing Officer and the Group Treasurer. Both Mr. Harrison and Dr. Dutton suggested to the Hospital Management Committee that there should be more delegation to them of matters of detail, but to no avail.

517. So far as we could discover there was no consideration of HM(68)28 commending greater delegation and fewer Subcommittees. Early in 1971 a member of the Management Committee submitted written proposals for simplifying the Subcommittee structure. It was decided to postpone discussion of these proposals until after the report of the Hospital Advisory Service had been received. That report said in paragraph 19 " The Committee structure is at present being reviewed " and recommended in paragraph 30.12 " The Hospital Management Committee should observe the advice given in HM(68)28— "Administration of Hospital Authorities "—in their review of the committee structure and the respective functions of the committee and its officers ". The Management Committee's subcommittee on the Hospital Advisory Service Report said " The H.M.C. feels that there is some need to re-examine the Subcommittee structure but as two Subcommittee chairmen were absent when this point was discussed, it will receive further consideration ". At the Management Committee meeting of 28 May it was decided to leave the Subcommittee structure discussion for another nine months. At the end of that nine months it was decided that there was no point in making any change before the reconstruction of the Health Service in 1974. Mr. Nichols told us that the matter was discussed by the Chairmen of the Subcommittees who were a kind of " inner cabinet ", and they decided that no changes were required. We understood from Mr. Nichols that the reason for keeping the four Subcommittees was that their existence helped to maintain regular visiting as members would visit the various hospitals after the business had been concluded. The alternative view that fewer meetings would leave more time for visiting had not been considered.

518. This catalogue of procrastination and unsound reasoning needs no further comment from us.

The representations from the Charge Nurses

519. On 27 November 1969 20 Charge Nurses at South Ockendon Hospital, calling themselves the Charge Nurses Association, wrote to the Secretary of State for Social Services, expressing concern about recent promotions in the

hospital of people not qualified as Registered Nurses for the Mentally Subnormal. " It is felt that if this trend is allowed to continue there is no incentive for the present holders of the R.N.M.S. certificate to remain here, or for students to continue their training ". They asked for clarification from the Management Committee of the criteria expected in regard to future promotions to " enable the staff to reach a decision as to whether it is in their interest to remain in the hospital or move on ". Copies of the letter were sent to the Chairman of the Management Committee, the Physician Superintendent, the Group Secretary and the Head of Nursing Services.

520. No meeting occurred between the Charge Nurses and the Management Committee or its Chairman until over four months later on 7 April, 1970. Mr. Nichols endeavoured to explain the delay. The correspondence, he said, followed discontent over a decision of the Establishments Subcommittee of which he was not a member. " I left it to the Secretary, Mr. Harrison, to pursue it, and as soon as we possibly could or when it was propitious a meeting was held. But I left it to the officers to make the necessary arrangements ". He agreed he could have had a meeting earlier if he had wished, but this, he explained, was an unrecognised organisation. " It is very difficult to ally yourself with an association of mushroom growth. Therefore, I looked to the Secretary to find out all the information he could ". This provoked the question " Mr. Nichols, here was a letter—forget it being a mushroom body—to the Secretary of State, signed by something like 18 of the charge nurses in the hospital expressing discontent. Now, that was a grave situation, was it not, calling, I suggest, for urgent action?" Mr. Nichols replied " I was sorry that this had come into being, but in the light of the information given me, I did not take this organisation seriously, and I think my judgment in the end has come to be right ".

521. We find the delay in meeting the Charge Nurses to be inexcusable. It indicates the same attitude of mind that had led to the Joint Consultative Committee with the staff falling into disuse during 1968. It started to meet again after the Board's Subcommittee, appointed after the death of Robert Robertson, had reported that it had not met for over 12 months and should be revived.

522. This Management Committee has badly needed an able Chairman with a fresh outlook on the problems of the hospital, and an injection of new members, with not only an ability to grasp the important factors in a situation, but also enquiring minds and the capacity to question previously accepted concepts. It was a mistake, as well as unfair, to have appointed Mr. Nichols as Chairman at his age with so many years on the Committee behind him.

Medical Staff and Standards

523. We have made a number of criticisms of Dr. Dutton and Dr. Harfst. We wish to put them into a proper and fair perspective.

Dr. Dutton

524. Dr. Dutton's ideas have been sound. He expresses himself well on paper. He was appointed a consultant psychiatrist for the Group in 1960. In January 1967 he was appointed Physician Superintendent for a term of five years. This was not renewed in January 1972, and he has continued as a consultant psychiatrist and has been appointed Chairman of the Medical Executive Committee.

For the first nine months of his time as Physician Superintendent he was the only consultant psychiatrist at South Ockendon Hospital. This was a very heavy work load for any man to carry even after he was joined by Dr. Harfst, and inevitably some parts of his work could not be done as well as he would have liked or as well as was required. Later they were joined by Drs. York-Moore and Hurst. It was the administrative aspects of Dr. Dutton's work which suffered. The fire and drive necessary to translate his ideas into a working policy and the necessary action were missing, as was the action necessary to correct mistakes. His laissez-faire approach left the good members of the staff free to experiment in their own way to the benefit of the hospital. But this approach, coupled with his over-high regard for the clinical autonomy of the other consultants, was in part responsible for a failure to correct and support the weak links which must always be present in any human structure. To all this there must be added the fact that Dr. Dutton has understandably become disenchanted by the contrast between the Department's proposals for the improvement of the subnormality services and the means provided to put them into practice.

525. So far as we have been able to discover nobody at any level has given sufficient guidance, or possibly thought, as to how the Cogwheel structure and the Salmon structure and multi-disciplinary teams are to operate in a subnormality hospital. How does one team relate to another? What becomes of the clinical autonomy of the consultant in a true multi-disciplinary framework? The real fault does not lie in the hospital. It lies with those who have substituted one system of medical administration for another with too little apparent recognition of the human elements and human problems involved, and the differences between, for example, an acute hospital and a subnormality hospital which provides the only home of many of its patients. The current language of " monitoring " and " modules " and the use of numbers rather than names to describe posts are all more appropriate to machines than people.

526. The problem of the changeover from one system to another will be overcome where the calibre of the people responsible for implementing it is high, not only in clinical skills, but also in the ability to think clearly and lay down a workable hospital policy. There is no reason to suppose that doctors are more likely to have this ability than anyone else, and it is unreal to imagine that it will always be supplied to the high degree necessary by management courses. The changeover from one system to another also needs a freshness and enthusiasm that will not always be found in this Cinderella branch of the National Health Service, and certainly was not present at South Ockendon Hospital. Whatever Dr. Dutton should have been called under the new system we are satisfied that he was regarded by all, including the Management Committee, as doing precisely the same job as he had as Physician Superintendent. It was unreal to have supposed otherwise, and this undoubtedly added to his problems. The Cogwheel multi-disciplinary structure that he introduced was to a large extent a paper one that failed to come to grips with the problems of the hospital. We have already seen in paragraphs 504–507 some of the odder features of this paper structure. Since the beginning of 1972 there has been a group multi-disciplinary team which meets about once every six months. The Medical Executive Committee and the Psychiatric Division meet at the same time every two to three months. We were unable to understand the relationship of these committees to each other, and Dr. Dutton agreed that it was to some extent a matter of chance to which committee a topic was referred. None of these committees or teams have considered

the problem villas of the hospital because they have been imbued with an anxiety not to appear to doubt the wisdom of the consultant or impinge on his clinical autonomy. We endeavour in Chapter X to suggest a more workable and easily understood multi-disciplinary framework for the hospital.

527. In December 1971 Dr. Dutton produced a document called an " operational policy " for the hospital. It was wrongly named. It sets targets for the future, but did not begin to provide an operational policy for making the best of the present with the resources available.

Dr. Harfst

528. Dr. Harfst is the consultant responsible for some of the hospital's problem villas, including Beech, Cypress and Willows. It was his first consultant's post and he needed support and guidance, in particular over Cypress. These he did not receive. The regime which he introduced into Cypress Villa was insensitive and inhumane, and his handling of the complaints flowing from it was inept. He is in our opinion a shy man who in the past has tended to adopt a rather forbidding demeanour to disguise his embarrassment and lack of security when dealing with critical parents. This has sometimes given an unfortunate impression. He appeared to us to be rather a solitary character, and we do not think that he found it easy to ask for help. Several charge nurses wrote to us expressing gratitude for the guidance and understanding he had given to them, and emphasising that Cypress had successes with very difficult patients when other villas had failed. We accept this as true. Before us his demeanour was initially rather cold and severe. But thereafter he was ready to admit faults and displayed a gentle charm and humour which would have achieved much with critical parents. We are sure that he is now far more ready and able to do the job required of him at South Ockendon than he was when he was appointed, and that working within a team he will succeed.

General medical care

529. Patients who were sufficiently ill to require transfer to the Gloucester Clinic received a very high standard of care. Those who were less ill and were nursed in their villas received a more variable standard. In Willows the standard of medical care was on occasions below that we would like to have seen. Nursing standards there were unacceptably low, and the medical supervision instead of lifting those standards appears to us sometimes to have accepted and adopted them.

Doctors on night duty

530. Doctors on night call are sometimes regular members of the medical staff who know the patients well and whose advice and support the nursing staff are always glad to receive. On other occasions they are general practitioners without any knowledge of the majority of the patients. We found that on at least one occasion the nursing staff hesitated to call such a doctor because they doubted whether any useful advice or treatment would be given, and this led to a decision not to call a doctor when one should have been called.

531. Whatever arrangements are made for the attendance of doctors at night it is important that there should be continuity and that the doctor should regard himself, and be treated, as an essential part of the medical staff serving the

hospital. He will thereby acquire knowledge of the patients and the staff who will in turn acquire confidence in him.

The Clinical Autonomy of Consultants

532. We have set out in considerable detail the views of both doctors and laymen on the nature and extent of the consultant's clinical autonomy. (See paragraphs 200 to 232.)

533. These views are unacceptable to us in the setting of South Ockendon Hospital which provides a semi-permanent home for many of its patients. No one person should be given or treated as having such power over the lives of the patients and be so free of any effective control. Consultants are as likely as anyone else to make mistakes or err in judgment, particularly when their work load is heavy and their resources inadequate. It is then that the support and guidance is needed.

534. We consider this problem further in Chapter X.

Nursing staff and standards of care

Senior Nursing Administration and Charge Nurses

535. Until 1967 nursing administration was divided on conventional lines between a Matron, and a Chief Male Nurse, Mr. Hubbard. When the Matron retired Mr. Searle was brought in and appointed Head of Nursing Services over Mr. Hubbard. On 1 July 1970 Mr. Andrews was appointed Chief Nursing Officer for the Group. He does not hold the R.N.M.S. certificate, which caused some resentment among the existing staff. In December 1971 Mr. Heffernan was appointed Principal Nursing Officer for South Ockendon Hospital. Mr. Searle and Mr. Hubbard did not apply for the post and are now Senior Nursing Officers each responsible for 11 villas. There was a long delay in introducing a Salmon structure in the Group, but this was eventually done in January 1972. These frequent changes must have been unsettling and have produced anxieties which for a time reduced the efficiency of the Nursing Administration.

536. When a new nursing structure is introduced into a Group it is necessary to strike a reasonable balance between the organisational requirements and the interests of staff. This was recognised by the National Nursing Staff Committee in their interim report of December 1968. They also recognised that " the senior posts in a Salmon structure involved new responsibilities and new duties. Inevitably not all existing staff will find it easy—or indeed possible—to adapt themselves fully to the changed roles which the new structure demands ". The Committee's recommendation to the Secretary of State, which he accepted, was that the top post in a new Salmon structure should be subject to open competition but that for posts below the top the emphasis should be on the absorption of the existing staff into the new Salmon graded posts. The March 1969 report of the Committee explained: " The reorganisation should not lead to staff whose performance has been of an acceptable standard being made redundant and unable to find comparable employment in other Groups. Therefore, existing staff should so far as possible be absorbed into their equivalent Salmon grade or, failing that, into the next lower Salmon grade on ' protective ' terms ".*

---

*Report by the National Nursing Staff Committee on the Selection and Appointment of Senior Nursing Staff in the Hospital Service, March 1969, paragraph 5.4.

537. We saw the results of this policy in the nursing management at South Ockendon Hospital. Mr. Andrews is introducing many changes for the better which are already bearing fruit. Mr. Heffernan's ambitions are enlightened and sound. On the other hand, the officers in middle management, senior nursing officers and unit officers, are not all of the calibre we would have wished. A Salmon structure gives increased opportunities and responsibilities to nurses. This increases the difficulties that arise if people are appointed to positions for which they are not fitted. In our view the duty of those making appointments should be first and foremost to the patients and to the members of the staff as a whole.

Charge Nurses

538. We were very pleased that a number of charge nurses came and gave evidence to us about their ambitions, the manner in which they have tried to achieve them, and their problems. They impressed and encouraged us. It is one of the strengths of the hospital that these imaginative nurses have been permitted to experiment and follow their own paths. With greater support they could have achieved still more. There were a few charge nurses who gave evidence before us whose attitudes we did not care for.

539. In our opinion one charge nurse should be made responsible for a villa, even though he will not be on duty both day shifts. At present no distinction in authority or responsibility is drawn between the charge nurse on the morning shift and the charge nurse on the afternoon shift.

Staff numbers

540. The present nursing establishment is 402 but it has not been revised since the reduction of the working week from 42 to 40 hours. Experience elsewhere suggests that it may be necessary to increase the establishment by 5% to allow for the reduction. The great need is to recruit more trained staff, but Table B in Appendix 3 shows that their numbers are declining rather than increasing. If they are recruited to the hospital in the future it can only be at the expense of other hospitals unless there is an appreciable increase in the numbers of qualified staff on which to draw.

541. The same table shows that there has been a marked increase in the number of unqualified staff. This is made up of 30 more student nurses, 3 more pupil nurses and the whole time equivalent of 24.6 more nursing assistants. We were informed that it would be difficult to increase the number of qualified staff without more accommodation at the hospital. Those now in the nurse training school will be unable to stay at the hospital after the completion of their training as there will be nowhere for them to live. The very staff therefore whom the hospital most needs are being driven elsewhere by shortage of accommodation. Expansion of the Nurse Training School is difficult when there is such a shortage of trained staff to supervise the students in the villas. We recommend that urgent consideration should be given to how much more staff accommodation is necessary.

542. South Ockendon Hospital lies about two miles outside the Metropolitan area which means that staff working in it are not entitled to the London Weighting of £126 per annum under the Whitley Council Scale. People living in the neighbourhood who want to nurse, and who might well work in South Ockendon

if the London Weighting applied, can obtain it by working in hospitals at Upminster, four miles away, or Romford, four miles away, or at Leytonstone House. This puts South Ockendon at a grave disadvantage in obtaining local staff. Efforts to get the London Weighting for the hospital have failed. We recommend that further consideration should be given to extending the London Weighting to this hospital. If it is again rejected the case for additional residential accommodation becomes even stronger than it already is.

543. We cannot leave the topic of staff recruitment without commenting on the numbers of ward nursing staff at South Ockendon Hospital who come from overseas. Some of these spoke reasonably good English but others had a poor grasp of the language. When certain of these nurses gave evidence we had great difficulty in understanding what they said and they in turn appeared not fully to understand the questions put to them. On visits to the wards also we met with difficulties of communication from the same cause. As we had difficulty, we can only assume that similar difficulty must arise in the giving and understanding of instructions by staff and the establishment of confidence between staff and patients. This is a most unsatisfactory situation. We understand that it is because sufficient staff cannot be found in this country that recruitment has to take place overseas in countries where the material standard of life is lower. We recommend that those concerned with the remuneration and conditions of service of nurses should be informed of this situation so that it may be given proper weight in their deliberations.

The standard of care

544. We have already said that most staff have done their best in difficult circumstances. The standard of care, however, has varied to a surprising degree from villa to villa. Although this has in part depended on the quality of the charge nurses, we observed that with a few exceptions the standard seemed lowest in the villas containing the most difficult patients. The significance of this must not be overlooked, for the proportion of severely disturbed patients in the hospital will inevitably increase as places elsewhere are found for those who no longer need hospital care.

545. The policy of concentrating difficult patients in certain villas, whatever the advantages to the hospital as a whole, has posed great problems for their staff who have not had the advantage of any clear hospital policy as to how they are to care for and train them. The more unresponsive the patients are to the staff's efforts at training the more encouragement and guidance the staff require. This has been lacking. In one villa, for example, we saw staff trying to occupy patients who had been divided into three groups, but they had very little idea of what they should have been trying to do. There is an obvious need for further guidance of staff in the use of play and other equipment. Some of the charge nurses and acting charge nurses were not making the best use of the staff under them. For example in one villa where more could have been done to occupy patients, two members of the nursing staff were turning down bedspreads in the middle of the afternoon. The absence of any clear policy or adequate guidance led in Willows Ward, for example, to some of the staff withholding cups of tea in order to teach good behaviour, while others, including the Charge Nurses thought that such means of training could never be justified. Such differing

139

views, in the absence of any policy, can only lead to confusion and must be bad for the patients.

546. The physical layout of many of the buildings, the shortage of baths and toilet arrangements are all barriers to high standards of care. In many villas the men are only shaved every other day. We heard evidence about queues of naked men waiting to be bathed. These are indignities which should not be accepted.

547. Unfortunately the hospital has to depend on student and pupil nurses to do much of the nursing. The General Nursing Council programme makes it necessary to move them from villa to villa about every eight weeks on average. This means they do not get to know the patients properly and adds to the difficulties of the charge nurses. These frequent changes are not in the interests of the patients or their relatives.

548. In our view an extended inservice training scheme at the hospital would do much to increase the standard of care. Visits to other hospitals or occasional attendance at lectures are better than nothing. In view of the increasing number of unqualified staff together with the need to acquaint all staff with modern concepts of care, what is required is a full-time inservice training officer. He will be responsible for organising courses covering these subjects. Staff will have to be released from duty in their villas for the duration of the course and the staff establishment should be revised to take this into account.

Use of side rooms and the control of violence

549. There is no hospital policy as to the circumstances in which or the duration for which a patient may be placed in seclusion. It has been left to each consultant to determine.

550. On 15 September 1970, Dr. Dutton wrote to all doctors working in the hospital asking them to " record in the case notes whenever a patient is placed in seclusion, the reasons for this and the duration of seclusion. Patients in side rooms must be visited by the ward doctors when doing the daily round and the fact entered in the patient's case notes ".

551. In September 1971 a day conference was held at the hospital on the " Guidelines for the Care of Patients Who Exhibit Violent Behaviour in Mental and Mental Subnormality Hospitals ". This was a consultative document prepared at the invitation of the National Association of Mental Health by a group of nurses, doctors and representatives of University Departments in consultation with the Royal College of Nursing, the Society of Mental Nurses, the General Nursing Council, the Association of Hospital Matrons, the National Association of Chief and Principal Nursing Officers, the Confederation of Health Service Employees, the Prison Officers' Association and the National Union of Public Employees. A copy was given to each of the hospital staff. It included the following proposals. " The use of physical methods of control, such as restraint or segregation, is only necessary when other methods have failed . . . Segregation should never be for a predetermined period which could be understood as a sentence, but only for as long as it may be necessary to calm the patient. In all emergencies the use of restraint should be therapeutic, never punitive. The test lies in the nurse's intention ' did he act in good faith for the benefit of the patient? ' . . . Whatever rules governing physical methods of control are adopted,

140

they should conform to a clearly stated policy discussed and approved at all levels of management. All patients, staff and members of the Hospital Management Committee should be aware of this Management Committee policy ".

552. The proposal that segregation should never be for a predetermined period appeared to conflict with Dr. Dutton's letter of 15 September 1970. We asked Dr. Dutton about this. To begin with he agreed there was a conflict and that some direction resolving it should have been issued. Later he said his letter could also mean that the time that a patient had been in the side room should be entered when he left it. This vacillation only emphasises the need for some policy to be laid down as proposed in the " Guidelines ". Dr. Dutton thought that a policy would best evolve by informal dissemination of discussion among the staff. We completely disagree.

553. These " Guidelines " were endorsed and developed in 1972 by a Liaison Committee formed by the Royal College of Psychiatrists and the Royal College of Nursing (Psychiatric Section). We support and endorse the committee's recommendations part of which are reproduced in Appendix 9. We know of no circumstances in which it would be right to depart from them.

554. The slapping of patients, however lightly, should never be permitted (see paragraphs 104 to 110).

Incontinence and habit training

555. In some villas, this has been pursued with vigour. The results have made all the work worthwhile. It is important that habit training should be urgently introduced in all villas where incontinence is a problem. The reduction of incontinence increases the dignity of patients and staff, in addition to lightening the work load.

Lay administration

556. Mr. Harrison, the Group Secretary, was appointed in May 1968 and took up his post in September 1968. He forms part of the Professional Executive Team which meets about once a fortnight. The other members are Dr. Dutton, the Chief Nursing Officer and the Group Treasurer. The subcommittee structure of the Management Committee and the attention of all the committees to matters of detail have made it impossible for Mr. Harrison and his colleagues to do their job as it should be done. More power must be delegated to them.

The handling of complaints

557. We dislike the word " complaint ". Unfortunately it has a stigma of disloyalty and dishonour attached to it which is deeply engrained at all levels in the hospital. South Ockendon Hospital, however, is not unique in this.

558. There is an unrealistic, unwise, and unhealthy reluctance to acknowledge that people are bound to make mistakes, and that people have a positive duty to comment upon matters that in their view should be put right. The person who " comments " or " complains " is too often made to feel that he is an outcast. We are satisfied that it needs a great deal of courage for a member of the staff to

" comment " on the way an individual carried out his or her work and that people who have shown the courage have too often had occasion to regret it. This is bad for the hospital.

559. We give some examples of these trends with some recommendations.

Complaints by patients about the staff

560. Sometimes a superficial investigation would be carried out at villa level, on others there would be no investigation of any kind. No complaint by a patient would get beyond villa level unless it was corroborated by a member of the staff or there were injuries which required explanation.

561. Mr. Shrimpton, a Senior State Enrolled Nurse, who has worked at the hospital since 1939 told us of an occasion in February 1968 when a patient in Beech told him that a charge nurse had hit another patient. He said " I took no notice ".

Q. " Because it was an allegation made by a patient ?" A. " That is right, yes ".

Q. " Just so we are absolutely clear, you are saying, Mr. Shrimpton, on no occasion when a patient said he had seen a member of the staff punch or hit somebody, on no occasion was anything ever done about it that you can remember? " A. " No, I do not think so, sir ".

Q. "And you would never even pass it on to the charge nurse? " A. " Well, I would if it was a bad case ".

562. In HM (66)15 the Minister of Health sent to hospitals procedure for investigating complaints by or on behalf of patients. It was, in our view, inappropriate for complaints by people suffering from mental handicap. In our view any complaints procedure for mentally handicapped people must include a duty on the member of staff to whom a complaint is made to record it forthwith in writing. It should be the duty of the charge nurse to transmit the complaint to the consultant and the unit nursing officer who would decide what steps to take in the light of current procedures or any new procedures which may be issued by the Department after receipt of the report of the Committee on Complaints under the Chairmanship of Mr. Michael Davies, Q.C. In our opinion, it is important that all such complaints and the action taken should be submitted in writing to the Group Secretary, the Chairman of the Medical Executive Committee, and the Chief Nursing Officer. The Group Secretary must keep the Chairman of the H.M.C. informed about complaints.

Complaints by patients and staff about staff

Charge Nurse Findlay's complaint

563. We set out the facts as we found them from the evidence of Mr. Findlay, Dr. Jones, Dr. Dutton, Mr. Searle, Mr. Balsdon, Mr. Laide and Dr. Harfst.

564. On 30 April 1968, Mr. Findlay, who had been working as a charge nurse in Cypress for about two weeks, made a written report to Dr. Harfst that patient WW (see paragraphs 183, 191 and 224) and another patient had accused another charge nurse of stealing their cigarettes and that Patient WW had also complained that he had stolen some of his money. On 1 May Patient WW asked to see Dr. Jones who found him in a very hysterical state and expressing fear that

the charge nurse would put him in the side room because he had accused him of stealing his cigarettes. Dr. Jones ordered him to be confined to the side room because of his disturbed state. The charge nurse against whom the allegation had been made entered in the ward report book for that day, but wrongly dated 2 May, that Patient WW had been " confined to side room with Dr. Harfst's permission for carrying tales about the staff ".

565. During the night Patient WW's behaviour was good. He asked to see Dr. Jones on the morning of 2 May and complained about being put in the side room and said that he thought he had been put there because he had made a complaint about the staff. Dr. Jones was informed by the staff that Patient WW had been found to have 40 cigarettes and 2 ounces of tobacco in his possession the night before. When Dr. Jones asked Patient WW about the allegation he refused to talk about it. Dr. Jones ordered his detention in the side room to continue. He was unable to give us any acceptable explanation for this.

566. On 3 May Dr. Dutton saw Patient WW, probably because Dr. Harfst went on holiday that morning,and ordered that Patient WW should remain in the side room until the following afternoon. Dr. Dutton must have known why Patient WW was in the side room.

567. Also on 3 May Mr. Pegley, a Deputy Chief Male Nurse, interviewed Mr. Findlay who told him that he had proof that cigarettes were missing from packets belonging to patients and that Mr. Turkington could give evidence about it. When Mr. Turkington was seen he denied any knowledge of the matter.

568. On a day, which is uncertain, very close to 3 May Dr. Jones asked Mr. Findlay to go over with him for an interview with Dr. Dutton. When he reached the Administration Block Mr. Findlay was seen by Mr. Searle, Mr. Pegley and Mr. Laide who conveyed their displeasure that he should have written to Dr. Harfst accusing a charge nurse of stealing cigarettes. They maintained that any such complaint should have been made through his nursing superiors. In the interview that followed with Dr. Dutton Mr. Findlay was upset and incoherent. Dr. Dutton used words which conveyed to him that he was wrong to waste his efforts on a patient of this calibre and that it could start an unfortunate precedent.

569. Dr. Dutton kept no note of the interview. Neither he nor any of Mr. Findlay's nursing superiors made any attempt to interview Mr. Findlay again when he was more composed. Nobody at any time took a written statement from Mr. Findlay. Nobody informed the Group Secretary or the Management Committee about the allegation. On the day of the interview with Dr. Dutton, Mr. Pegley and Mr. Searle removed Mr. Findlay from further duty on Cypress as from the following morning, although he was due to go on holiday very shortly. We are satisfied that he was moved from Cypress in order to humiliate him and deter him from passing on similar complaints by patients in future. We heard no evidence that justified keeping Patient WW in a side room for one hour, let alone four days. The investigation of the complaint was inadequate. Mr. Findlay was made to feel a traitor. As a result of this episode the fears of patients and staff about the consequences of making or passing on complaints must have been intensified.

570. We did not investigate whether the charge of theft was well founded as the charge nurse against whom the allegation was made was not able to give evidence to us about it.

143

Complaints by Staff about Staff

Sister T's complaint

571. On 30 January 1969 Sister T reported to Dr. Benton that patients had been slapped by members of the staff in Redmayes Villa between April and December 1968. She was interviewed by Dr. Dutton and said that she had reported the incidents to other staff. All these staff except one denied having been told about the incidents. The exception, who was an Assistant Matron, agreed that Sister T had reported a slapping incident but maintained that the allegation was so vague that she had done nothing about it. One of the staff against whom slapping had been alleged admitted this had occurred.

572. When Dr. Dutton reported these events to the Chairman and Vice-Chairman of the Management Committee he omitted to mention that the Assistant Matron agreed that Sister T had reported a slapping incident but she had done nothing about it.

573. Disciplinary proceedings were brought not only against the nurse who admitted slapping two patients but also against Sister T for failing to make written reports of the incidents at the time they occurred. Both were censured. No disciplinary charge was preferred against the Assistant Matron.

574. We consider that this was a most unfortunate episode which was likely to deter other staff from having second thoughts and reporting matters which they should have reported earlier. It required courage to make the allegations at all, and Sister T should not have been censured for her earlier failure to make a written report. We can see no reason for distinguishing between Sister T and the Assistant Matron.

575. We have already referred to the failure to take any disciplinary action against Mr. Large over his failure, revealed by his own version of events, to take proper care of Robert Robertson or make out the accident report properly or make a proper report to Dr. Jones. (See paragraphs 127 to 130.)

576. We feel that there is a tendency to give undue support to people who are or should be justly criticised. Mr. Searle has written glowing references for Mr. Large since the death of Robert Robertson. The notice of discontinuance of training by Mr. Powell after the assault on GG should not have stated that his conduct was " satisfactory on all counts ".

Parents

577. We found that parents who are critical of the way their children are cared for are resented by many of the nursing staff, and, indeed, by some of the medical staff. The attitude is prevalent " If they can't manage their child themselves why criticise us when we have so many more to try to care for? " This has on occasions led to nurses saying " If you don't like it you can always take him (or her) home ". Inservice training and ward meetings should cover this kind of problem. We have already mentioned that changes in staff impose strains not only on the patients and other staff but also on parents who are constantly having to forge new bonds of goodwill and understanding.

Catering

578. In the written and oral evidence we received there were only a few comments on the catering. Patients and their relatives seemed on the whole to be satisfied with the food. One relative wrote:

" The food is good, adequate and there appears to be a variety. D— always tells me she has enjoyed her dinner ".

579. In 1971, the cost per week per patient of food alone was £1·75 which was 10p above the national average for hospitals for the mentally handicapped, and the weekly cost has since risen to £2·12 a head.

580. The Group Secretary in his evidence said that the Hospital Management Committee was conscious of some weaknesses in the catering arrangements. Whilst the quantity of food was considered adequate its quality was sometimes criticised. The kitchen was originally designed for a hospital half the present size of South Ockendon Hospital and the distribution of food also presented a problem because of the size and layout of the villas. This latter problem had been partly met by introducing a system of heated trolleys. It had been very difficult to recruit an adequate number of qualified cooking staff of the right calibre. Service in the wards had to be by the nursing staff because there were inadequate numbers of domestic staff, and they were not trained. We were told that the Board were considering a small capital scheme aimed at improving the kitchen and the staff dining room in 1972/73.

581. We ourselves did not much like the food when we lunched in Poplars Ward. We also thought that the service of meals should have been made to seem less institutional. We must record, however, that the helpings were generous and were eaten rapidly and with apparent satisfaction by our table companions. The charge nurse told us that normally the meals were better than on that day.

582. The mother of a patient who gave evidence to us is herself a dietician praised the food given to patients who were unable to chew, and the care taken in providing all the necessary vitamins for such patients.

583. There is room for improvement in the catering arrangements, and the hospital authorities are clearly aware of this. We hope that they will succeed in overcoming the difficulties which at present prevent a better service from being provided.

Laundry

584. Here again the hospital authorities are conscious of weaknesses in the service available. The difficulties are much the same as for catering—inadequate space and equipment and difficulty in recruiting suitable staff. A scheme of improvements is, we were told, in the Board's current programme.

585. The inadequacy of the laundry is one of the reasons why patients are not yet able normally to wear their own clothing or personal clothing provided by the hospital, as is the Department's policy. Personal laundering of the varied materials now commonly used cannot be coped with in a laundry designed for processing large quantities of items in bulk. Space is needed for proper checking and classification of the clothing received and later for packing and despatching it. Different types of machines are needed for washing, drying and finishing the

garments. A considerable amount of work is involved in the wards also in marking each item of clothing and checking that it is returned. Detailed advice was issued to hospital authorities by the Department of Health and Social Security in April 1972 on the best ways of dealing with this problem, and we hope that the Hospital Management Committee and the Regional Hospital Board will give urgent attention to the matter. The wearing of personal clothing, properly fitting, is in our view one of the essential factors in providing a dignified and homelike environment for long-stay patients.

Contribution of Local Authorities

586. The South Ockendon Group receives patients from areas with a total population of some 1,600,000 lying within the boundaries of 12 local authorities (Herts and Essex County Councils, Southend County Borough, eight London Boroughs and the City). Admissions from the whole catchment area are normally to South Ockendon Hospital or Leytonstone House Hospital; no hospital is linked solely to any one part of the catchment area.

587. Co-operation with so large a number of authorities is difficult, and particularly so in a situation where the hospitals, for lack of beds, are unable to admit patients requiring hospital care, and where the local authorities, for lack of residential homes, are unable to accept from the hospital those patients who could be returned to the community.

588. In 1966 an assessment by the hospital staff suggested that 127 patients in the South Ockendon Group were not in need of hospital care. Names of these patients were sent to the local authorities concerned and by the end of the year 66 had been acknowledged by the local authorities as suitable for community care, the rest being still under discussion. Yet, after considerable correspondence, only three of these patients were actually discharged because the local authorities concerned could not make suitable provision for the others. At the same time, there was a waiting list of over 200 people seeking admission to hospital in the South Ockendon Group.

589. In March 1969 the Hospital Management Committee, with the support of the Board and the Secretary of State, placed a ban on all admissions to South Ockendon Hospital (other than the security unit in Cypress Villa). This lasted until July 1970 when, after discussions between the Board and the Group it was agreed to institute a policy of 1 admission for every 4 discharges. This 1 : 4 admission rate has continued to operate with a resultant decrease in the numbers of hospital patients. However, in an effort to help families caring for mentally handicapped persons, some beds were made available for short-term admissions. This has resulted in 23 patients admitted for short-term care becoming permanent residents, thus jeopardising the policy of reducing the number of patients in the overcrowded hospital. Local authorities for their part have found themselves unable to gain admission to South Ockendon Hospital for residents assessed by their consultant adviser as in need of hospital care. One London Borough complained that it had been obliged to place its residents elsewhere at the expense of the authority.

590. We invited the 12 local authorities whose boundaries lay wholly or partly within the catchment area of the South Ockendon Group to supply information

about their present provision and future plans for the care of the mentally handicapped. All accepted this invitation. Details of the places available in their residential homes are given in Appendix 10. Four of the authorities at present have no homes at all and six others have none for children. All except one authority have plans for providing at least one home within the next two years. Herts and Essex County Councils each plan to provide two or three homes a year for the next ten years. But in all areas the new homes are likely to be used first to relieve families rather than to take patients from hospital, and it will probably be some years before they have a substantial effect on the relief of overcrowding in hospitals.

591. Witnesses on behalf of the Board declared with some vehemence that the advice given to local authorities in Cmnd. 4683 would not in itself prove sufficient to ensure the rapid increase in local authority provision of residential homes which was needed. They believed that there should in each area be joint planning of the hospital and community needs of the mentally handicapped, and that the Department of Health and Social Security itself should take an active part both in planning and in giving guidance; above all the central Government should provide special financial aid to the local authorities. Cmnd. 4683 (paragraphs 268 and 269) asked each Board to have detailed discussions with each of the local authorities in its region and to produce co-ordinated plans for each area. We endorse this request and hope that the Department will support Boards and local authorities in this joint planning exercise.

592. The replies from the 12 local authorities showed that their Social Service Departments had made provision with varying degrees of adequacy for the non-residential care of their mentally handicapped residents. Particulars of the adult training centre places available and planned are given in Appendix 10, and show that every authority has at least one centre and that 6 out of 11* have plans to increase their provision. At least half of the local authorities were giving less social work support to the families of mentally handicapped residents than they thought desirable, and several mentioned the limitations imposed upon them by the shortage of social workers.

593. Despite the difficulties resulting from lack of accommodation, geography and the large number of local authorities relying on the South Ockendon Group for hospital services for the mentally handicapped, considerable effort has been made to achieve and maintain good liaison between the hospital and local authorities and their staff at all levels. Professor Ramsay said that during his term as Senior Administrative Medical Officer he had had regular contacts with all the Medical Officers of Health in the Region. As soon as the new Social Service Directors were appointed in 1971 he sponsored a series of meetings with them to which the Medical Officers of Health were also invited. The Hospital Management Committee has the benefit of two Medical Officers of Health (Essex and Southend) among their members. Relations between consultants of the hospital and the local authorities are generally good. Each of the 12 local authorities has been given the name of the consultant psychiatrist on the staff of South Ockendon Hospital responsible for their area. Some of the local authorities make full use of the consultant service and this has proved invaluable

*The City of London explained that all mental health work for the City is carried out on an agency basis by the London Borough of Tower Hamlets.

in determining admissions, discharges and positive therapeutic measures. Other authorities have not yet made full use of this service. As a matter of policy as well as convenience arrangements have been made for outpatient clinics to be held regularly in the premises of seven of the local authorities as well as at South Ockendon, Leytonstone House and the Eastern Hospital: this has enabled the consultants to develop close links with local authority social workers, teachers in the new Special Schools and staff in the adult training centres. Several of the local authorities who wrote to us mentioned with appreciation an excellent relationship with the consultant for their area and the value of his advice on the care of mentally handicapped people in the community. Some local authorities spoke also of very close liaison between their social workers and the South Ockendon Hospital, but others complained of a shortage of social work staff that made co-operation very difficult.

Reduction of Overcrowding since March 1971 and in the Future

594. We dealt with the growth of overcrowding in paragraphs 11 and 30 to 35 and with the steps to deal with it between February 1969 and March 1971 in paragraphs 134 to 152.

595. By June 1972 the number of patients in residence had been reduced to 906. On average the patients in the hospital have the minimum night space of 50 square feet and the minimum day space of 30 square feet which the Secretary of State laid down in 1969 as an interim target for achievement in the years 1970–75 but four wards are still below this standard for both day and night space and six wards are below the standard either in day space or in night space. The interim target of reducing the numbers in adult wards below 50 and those in childrens' wards below 30 will be achieved during 1973. It is vital to remember, however, that as long ago as 1960 the Ministry of Health laid down a standard of 60 square feet night space per patient, and in 1965 HM(65)104 stated "A ward should not normally accommodate more than 30 adult patients or 20 children ". The staff at the hospital say that it is essential that the numbers should be reduced to these levels without delay in the low grade wards if they are to do the job of training which they are taught, and which is now rightly expected of them. We entirely agree: the 1969 " interim measures " are in our opinion inappropriate, even as minimum standards, for such villas as Beech.

596. We were told that the target of reducing the maximum numbers in wards to 30 adults and 20 children each of whom will have 70 square feet night space and 48 square feet day space will be achieved during 1975 if the Board's building programme throughout the region proceeds according to plan. The position should be reviewed to ensure that at least Beech and Poplars achieve these standards during 1973. One way of achieving this may be the provision of small units in which the very disturbed patients can be cared for with a much higher staff ratio.

597. In September 1972 the medical and nursing staff of South Ockendon Hospital undertook a further survey of patients to assess their fitness to be discharged to live in residential homes. They decided that 294 of the patients would be fit for discharge if care could be provided for them in the community. The standards were different from those used in 1966 and the assessment has not yet been agreed with all the local authorities concerned.

CHAPTER X

THE CREATION OF A HOME

598. We take as the theme of this chapter two of the general principles set out in paragraph 40 of Better Services for the Mentally Handicapped (Cmnd. 4683).

" When a handicapped person has to leave his family home, temporarily or permanently, the substitute home should be as homelike as possible, even if it is also a hospital ".

" There should be a proper co-ordination in the application of relevant skills for the benefit of individual handicapped people and their families, and in the planning and administration of relevant services, whether or not these cross administrative frontiers ".

We like the repetition of the word " home ". We hope that it will continue to be used and believe that its use will help to promote and maintain right thinking and action.

What are the ingredients of a home for mentally handicapped people?

Firstly there must be a building in which to spend that part of the day which is not occupied by outside work or leisure activities.

599. There should be reasonable privacy. If a number of people have to live in one building they will want to sleep in small groups if they cannot have rooms of their own. Large dormitories with lines of beds are the antithesis of home. Where they exist they should be subdivided. Patients using lavatories should not be exposed to the gaze of other people. Decoration and furnishing should be comparable to that found in other homes throughout the land. Standardisation should be avoided. Rows of hospital type beds are unnecessary and unhomely.

Secondly, there must be a homely way of life.

600. This means

i. *There must be people who will provide throughout the day and night homemaking care and attention needed by those living there and looked for by their relatives and friends.*

This care and attention covers many activities which go far beyond purely medical or nursing skills. If the aim is truly to create a home these activities will be at least as important as the purely medical and nursing aspects of the work. Mr. Campanella, who is the charge nurse in Poplars Villa, described his job in a letter to a local paper in this way " My role?—father figure, organiser, counsellor, entertainer, handyman, provider, secretary to myself and patients, adviser to parents, teacher to my juniors, beggar and collector of secondhand clothes and furniture for the ward. As you see the list is unending. The same can be said for every single member of the staff ".

ii. What is comprehended by Mr. Campanella's " father (and we add ' mother ') figure? " Someone who will guide and develop character.

Someone who will teach independence. Someone to see that the occupant is properly clothed. Someone to nurse him when ill. Someone to call a doctor when one is needed. Someone to enlist skilled teachers when they are necessary. The list is indeed unending.

  iii. *There must be work and occupation, entertainments and outings, and the coming and going of friends.*

  iv. Without these our own homes would become prisons. We would become frustrated, inward looking, difficult people, and would require more frequent treatment from our doctors.

  v. The organisations referred to in Chapter VIII endeavour to provide all these essentials of home life.

  vi. *There must be skilled medical attention when this is necessary and adequate dental and physiotherapy and speech therapy services.*

601. In summary, therefore, it is the caring staff working in the villas who create the home and form the hub round which its life revolves. They are assisted by the medical and paramedical services who provide their own specialist knowledge when it is needed, and by the many voluntary workers.

602. All these aspects of home making and support overlap and complement each other. Those responsible for their provision must work together as a multi-disciplinary team.

603. We have already referred to the apparent contradiction between a multi-disciplinary approach to the care of patients and the interpretation put on the autonomy of the consultant by the Board, the Hospital Management Committee, Dr. Dutton and the other consultants at the hospital.

604. We believe that membership of a multi-disciplinary team involves each individual submerging his or her individual professional identity in pursuit of the common goal. Such an approach need not conflict with the individual responsibility of consultants in strictly clinical matters, and we strongly agree with the view expressed elsewhere* that present day psychiatry is multi-disciplinary in its nature.

605. The success of the team will depend on the quality of the relationship and rapport that is established between members. This will be governed by the personality, experience and skill of each person. Some teams will perform well, some adequately and some badly. It is therefore essential in our opinion that multi-disciplinary teams operating at unit level should be subject to supervision *and* correction within the hospital. This, we consider, must be provided by another multi-disciplinary team and not by individual disciplines.

A possible Multi-disciplinary Framework for the Hospital

A Hospital Multi-disciplinary Team consisting of medical, nursing and other professional representatives

606. The role of this team would be

  i. to translate the guidance from the Department, Board and Group into

---

*Second Report of the Joint Working Party on the Organisation of Medical Work in Hospitals: paragraph 7.11.

a working policy of care for each villa in the hospital asking always what do the patients need if this hospital is to be a home. This will involve deciding how to make the best use of inadequate resources and the fixing of priorities, which in turn will mean identifying the real problem areas in the hospital.

ii. to see that the working policy it lays down is put into practice or modified as necessary. This again will involve scrutiny of the standard of overall care in villas and directions for improvement where this is necessary. The team will probably consider in turn each of the villas starting with the most difficult. We emphasise that a working policy must include not only plans for future improvements but also plans to make the best possible use of the limited human and material resources available.

607. The Hospital Multi-disciplinary Team should elect a chairman to ensure some continuity. It is not necessary in our opinion that he should be a doctor. What is necessary is that he should be a good chairman who preferably has no particular axe to grind or hobby horse to ride. The team should meet at least once a month.

608. This team will be doing part of the job that the Management Committee should have been doing. It will be even more important after April 1974 as we do not see how District Management Teams will have the time or knowledge to deal with these problems. Its line of communication upwards will be with the Group Professional Executive, which at present consists of the Chairman of the Medical Executive Committee, Group Secretary, Chief Nursing Officer and Treasurer, until April 1974, and thereafter with the District Management Team

609. It is essential that there is adequate secretarial and office help for this team. Much information will have to be collected and prepared for its members, full minutes will have to be kept, and information will have to be sent to the villas.

610. Committees or meetings of separate disciplines will continue to be necessary from time to time. But we can see no need in this Group for both a Medical Executive Committee and a Psychiatric Division. They should be amalgamated in name as well as in fact. Medical Executive Committees in psychiatric groups generally include all consultants, since they are few in number. It is not possible to lay down any hard and fast line on matters which should go to purely medical or nursing meetings. The essential thing to keep in mind is that it is the Hospital Multi-disciplinary Team which blends the thoughts of the separate disciplines so as to achieve a homelike way of life and care for the patients. The separate disciplines will no doubt meet from time to time to see whether there are problems with which the Hospital Multi-disciplinary Team are failing to grapple or matters it is failing to take into account. On other occasions matters will be referred by the Hospital Multi-disciplinary Team to the individual disciplines for discussion and recommendation and action.

The Activities Team

611. This will consist of the Activities Officer, the Head of Occupational Therapy, the Recreations Officer and the Voluntary Work Organiser.

612. This team will be concerned with organising to the best advantage and further developing all the activities dealt with in Chapter VIII.

613. It will be responsible to the Hospital Multi-disciplinary Team and will work through its own members and through the Unit Multi-disciplinary Teams considered below. When it considers a particular villa it will no doubt invite staff from that villa to attend its meeting.

614. We have already said that much of the work done in the Activities Centre and in the Occupational Therapy building appears similar. We suggest that the occupational therapist should concentrate on the patients who really need her highly trained professional skill, and that nursing staff, at present under Mr. Wood, continue to expand the work they are doing with the great mass of the patients. If the occupational therapist is seen as the specialist who concerns herself with those patients who can gain most from her special training, she and her department will be seen in their true position as part of the Activities Team.

615. This team will probably need to meet weekly. Once again it is essential that there is adequate secretarial and office help. This will free the members to do their proper work. Agenda and Minutes of its meetings should be sent to all members of the Hospital Multi-disciplinary Team.

Unit Multi-disciplinary Teams

616. Each unit will adopt a multi-disciplinary approach to its work. The basic team will be the unit nursing officer, nursing representatives from the villas, members of the medical staff and a representative from the Activities Team; but membership of the team will contract, expand or vary according to the matters to be discussed, which will cover every aspect of the patients' needs. Sometimes the team will consider problems common to all the villas in the unit: at others it may deal with the affairs of just one villa. One meeting a month will probably be sufficient.

617. These teams will be responsible to the Hospital Multi-disciplinary Team and should send their minutes to that team, the Administration, and the Principal Nursing Officer and the Senior Nursing Officer responsible for the unit.

618. Every effort should be made to ensure that a unit nursing officer has one consultant dealing with all the villas in his unit. This will result in saving of time and may in some cases make it easier for all the staff in a unit to reach agreement on a common approach to their work.

619. At villa level more frequent meetings will take place—sometimes villa staff meetings—sometimes case conferences—sometimes gatherings of parents and voluntary workers. We suggest that these should be less formal and that there should be no need for minutes. We suggest that when a case conference discusses a particular patient the notes should be put in the medical file of that patient. At present they appear to be entered only in a ward book.

620. If the best is to be obtained from these teams it is again important that there should be adequate secretarial help. Lay people can do much of the administrative work which will be involved and leave the trained personnel to do their work. The more homelike a villa becomes the more secretarial work there will be; for example, making arrangements for shopping expeditions, visits to

places of interest and other outings, the organisation of parents' associations, villa open days, and so on. This kind of help need not be full time but it should be paid. We believe that it will attract people living in the locality who do not want to nurse, and that these people will form useful links with the surrounding population which may also increase staff recruitment all round. The right kind of person would be drawn fully into all aspects of villa life.

621. This is only a suggested multi-disciplinary structure for the hospital. It should be modified as appropriate and should at all times be flexible and sensitive to changing needs. The vital thing in our view is that each Unit Multi-disciplinary Team should be responsible to and subject to direction by a Hospital Multi-disciplinary Team, and that the teams should be concerned with all aspects of care. We consider that the unit teams should have a great deal of freedom in applying the policy laid down by the Hospital Multi-disciplinary Team, but the power must exist within the hospital, and where necessary, be used to correct aspects of care that are going wrong.

622. It should in our opinion be the responsibility of the Chairman of the Medical Executive Committee to discuss with a consultant any problems of which he is aware within the strictly clinical field of that consultant and to urge a change of policy where he feels this desirable. If he is unable to achieve a satisfactory solution he must formally inform the Senior Administrative Medical Officer of the position.

623. We believe that the more homelike becomes the way of life in hospital the greater will become the proportion of patients who confound earlier expectation and reach a stage when they are ready to return to their own homes. Very often, however, there will be no home available. Hostels must be provided for such patients as a matter or urgency. Nothing can be more disheartening for staff and patients than to find that the means of final rehabilitation are denied. If the present building programme is so limited by finance that hostels are unlikely to be provided for more than a very few patients now in hospital for some years we feel that it is important that this should be brought clearly to the public's attention. Public opinion can bring about changes. Likewise voluntary organisations or individuals can only step in and provide the necessary facilities when they know the extent of the need and the time for which it is likely to remain unmet by the National Health Service.

1974

624. We must refer to the possible impact on South Ockendon Hospital of the reorganisation of the National Health Service which is due to take place in April 1974. The proposed Community Health Councils have a potential for good, but they also carry obvious dangers for the hospital.

625. We have seen in this report how those who feel themselves criticised, particularly by those who they feel do not understand, close ranks against the critics, sometimes to an extent that they are defending the indefensible. The lower the calibre of the management the more likely this is to occur. We fear that unless a very careful watch is kept the District Management Team and the Health Council may remain at arms' length, and that the Management Team will speedily resent a Health Council that is doing its work. Criticism by the Health Council of the hospital could also lead to a similar situation.

626. The Community Health Councils may well remain ignorant of undesirable aspects of care in a hospital. There may be a tendency for District Management Teams, who will be extremely busy, to assume that all is well where the public watchdog is silent.

627. In order to reduce these dangers at South Ockendon Hospital we suggest that some people should be appointed to the Council because of their existing interest and work in the hospital. We have in mind some members of the League of Friends who know the staff and have been actively concerned in creating homelike conditions. The South Ockendon League of Friends certainly has some members of the right calibre. We feel that an opportunity would be lost if the Health Councils were composed mainly of former Management Committee members.

628. 1974 also causes us this additional concern. The new District Management Team will understandably be working towards new concepts of care based on much smaller hospitals serving a district. South Ockendon will for years have more patients than current thinking considers desirable. It will have to serve several districts. There is a danger that it will be regarded as an unfortunate but unavoidable anachronism eating up money which should be used to introduce more up-to-date methods of care. Any such attitude may adversely affect the money allocated to it. In our opinion the site and layout of the buildings at South Ockendon have a considerable potential. The surroundings are pleasant. It is not too remote from outside communities although its present catchment area is too wide.

CHAPTER XI
CONCLUSIONS AND RECOMMENDATIONS

Conclusions

629. South Ockendon Hospital has a higher than average proportion of severely handicapped patients (29). In 1968, the space available for these patients in wards and departments and the numbers of nursing staff employed to care for them were seriously inadequate and they have remained so, to a decreasing extent, in subsequent years (28–29).

630. We find that at least three patients, whose histories are related, suffered a deterioration in their condition because of the effects of overcrowding, staff shortage and lack of facilities. The complaints of the parents of these three patients were justified. During the last two years there has been some improvement in the condition of these patients; in two cases, improvement followed transfer to Little Highwood Hospital (Chapter III).

Beech Villa

631. In 1968 and 1969, Beech Villa was overcrowded and understaffed. There was very frequent violence involving attacks by patients on other patients and staff (61).

Patient GG

632. During the night of 16 to 17 June 1968, patient GG received injuries to his arms, legs, back, buttocks and lower abdomen, mainly weals and punctate wounds, which could have been caused by a bath brush which was kept at night in a locked bathroom to which only the staff had a key.

633. We find that Mr. Powell, a student nurse then aged 19, who was in charge of the ward that night took part in an assault on patient GG which caused the injuries found and that this assault was probably committed because GG had wetted his bed. We are unable to say whether the other member of the staff who was on duty, Mr. Ramen, a nursing assistant, took part in the assault because he has gone abroad and he did not give evidence. (65–79).

634. We consider that Beech Villa should not have been left in charge of two young and inexperienced nurses. (80).

635. We find that the disciplinary proceedings taken by the Hospital Management Committee were unsatisfactory in that they charged both nurses with negligence but did not specify the acts or omissions upon which the charge of negilence was based (82).

636. We find that Mr. Hubbard was gravely inaccurate when, in notifying the General Nursing Council of Mr. Powell's discontinuance of training, he indicated that his conduct had been " satisfactory on all counts " (84).

Allegations made by Mr. Crowson

637. We accept Mr. Crowson's evidence that, on the morning of 20 February 1969 between about 6.45 and 7.00 a.m., he saw three separate incidents in which Mr. Large struck patient HH across the face with a folded sheet to wipe his nose: kicked patient CC in the face with the sole of his shoe to stop him chewing and tearing a drawsheet: and struck patient DD with the side of his hand. None of the assaults was sufficiently serious to have left marks visible on examination about 55 hours later. (92 to 98).

638. We find that there was inadequate counselling of staff on methods of dealing with disturbed patients (110). Such guidance would have reduced the risk of assaults of the kind which Mr. Crowson witnessed on 20 February 1969 (92) and which he himself committed on another occasion (101) and would have prevented the slapping of patients acknowledged by other witnesses (104 to 108).

Death of Patient Robert Robertson

639. At about 3.15 p.m. on 20 February 1969, Robert Robertson, a subnormal patient, aged 38, who suffered from epilepsy and had a schizophrenic personality, died from internal injuries which were revealed by post mortem examination.

640. We find that
   a. Mr. Large saw Robert Robertson being aggressive to another patient, probably JJ, between 7.00 and 7.45 a.m. and it was for this reason he pulled him struggling into the low grade room.
   b. Mr. Large's evidence that he saw JJ stamping on Robert Robertson was untrue. Our reasons for rejecting this evidence are
      i. nothing that Mr. Large said or wrote before going off duty referred to his having seen Robert Robertson being jumped or stamped on.
      ii. it is in our opinion inconceivable that he would have failed to mention this jumping or stamping both in the injury report and in his discussion with Dr. Jones, had it occurred.
      iii. when taking Robert Robertson to the low grade room, Mr. Large told Mr. Maghoo that he had been aggressive and he was still behaving an in aggressive manner. It is highly improbable that Robert Robertson would have been struggling then if he had immediately before been stamped or jumped on with sufficient force to cause the internal injuries described by Dr. Whitehead. (119–121).

641. We are unable to reach any sure conclusion on the manner or circumstances in which Robert Robertson received the injuries from which he died and we are satisfied that no other enquiries or proceedings would enable a sure conclusion to be arrived at (122).

642. No-one connected with the hospital considered the question whether Mr. Large's own version of events revealed him as unfit to continue as a charge nurse. We find that on Mr. Large's account of the events of the morning, his care of Robert Robertson was inadequate when measured against what he claimed to have seen, as was also his failure to record in the injury report or to tell Dr. Jones of the stamping that he alleged had occurred. There were failures

to take action by the Group's senior medical nursing and administrative staff and failure by the HMC to notice this omission and to initiate action (127 and 129–130).

643. We find that it was known to responsible officers at the Regional Hospital Board and to Dr. Dutton that Dr. Jones had signed the injury report without examining patient Robert Robertson, but no-one spoke to Dr. Jones about this and no steps were taken to ensure that this did not happen on other occasions until Dr. Dutton sent out an instruction in September 1972 (133).

Events Resulting from the Death of Robert Robertson

644. Between 1969 and 1971, reports on the position at South Ockendon Hospital were made by a sub-committee of the Regional Hospital Board, by the Post-Ely Policy Working Party's Visiting Team and by the Hospital Advisory Service. All agreed that the overcrowding, staff shortage and inadequate facilities needed urgent remedial action (135 to 141).

645. During the same period the number of patients was reduced by about 85 as a result of a ban on admissions (except to the security unit) from March 1969 until July 1970, followed by a policy of 1 admission to 4 discharges, and the transfer of 50 patients to Little Highwood Hospital in January 1971. A prefabricated unit was erected in order to provide accommodation for patients while existing villas were upgraded (148 and 150).

646. We find that these measures improved the situation in the hospital but left it still far from satisfactory. We recognise, however, that the pressure from the community to resume admissions in July 1970 was very great and that so long as the ban on admissions remained in force there would be families who would suffer very great hardship (151).

Allegation of Mr. Hill

647. We find that Mr. Hill's allegation of ill-treatment of a patient is not substantiated (155).

Beech Villa today

648. We find that the reduction in the number of patients to 40 and the efforts made to brighten the building and train the patients have improved this villa. Nevertheless it remains unattractive and lacking in comfort (154).

649. We consider that the gathering together in one villa of so large a number of disturbed patients makes improvement of their condition more difficult (161, 545).

Cypress Villa

Planning and operation up to September 1967

650. We find that Dr. Dutton ran the security unit in Cypress Villa as it should have been run subject to only two criticisms:
   a. the compulsory seclusion of all new patients in a side room for two days was undesirable and unnecessary except where a patient arrived in a disturbed state and

b. the administrative inconvenience of allowing patients to wear private clothing was not sufficient justification for his instruction forbidding this. (172–176)

Changes introduced by Dr. Harfst

651. We find that the RHB should have given greater guidance on policy to Dr. Harfst (180).

652. We find that Dr. Harfst quickly introduced a change of policy under which Cypress became a villa of maximum security from which patients were no longer taken out for occupational or industrial therapy or for recreation and in which side rooms were used in a punitive manner (177–187). He arranged for structural changes to the building (188–189) and introduced strict rules on security for the guidance of staff (190).

653. We find in particular that:
   a. every patient admitted to Cypress was confined in a side room and deprived of all reasonable comforts for an average of seven days. Subsequently seclusion in side rooms was ordered for punitive purposes, sometimes for as much as four weeks (192).
   b. before long, the furniture in side rooms consisted of only a mattress on the floor. There was neither locker nor chair. Patients were clothed only in pyjamas, with the cord removed from the trousers (193).

654. We find that Dr. Harfst's memorandum of February 1969 which was circulated to the Management Committee members clearly set out his policy on maximum security, but no objection to it was raised by the HMC (194 to 196).

The effect of clinical autonomy

655. We find that until after September 1969 when the mother of patient S made complaints about the treatment of her son, no criticism of the regime in Cypress Villa was made by the RHB, the HMC or any of their officers, although the villa had been visited by the Chairman, Senior Administrative Medical Officer and Secretary of the RHB and by the Chairman and Vice-Chairman of the HMC. This was because all concerned were reluctant to appear to call a consultant's decision into question (200 to 232).

656. We find that even when Dr. Dutton, as Physician Superintendent, investigated some of the complaints by the mother of patient S and discovered things that were not acceptable to him he did not express this opinion either to Dr. Ramsay or to the HMC (223).

657. In our view, the following action should have been taken:—
   a. before the villa opened and again when Dr. Harfst joined the hospital, Dr. Dutton should have convened a multi-disciplinary meeting to discuss the kind of patient to be admitted, the kind of care and treatment that should be provided, the manner in which the villa would be run, the equipment required and how any problems foreseen would be overcome. A clear policy directive should have been worked out and written down.
   b. the senior officers of the group should have provided, and the Management Committee members should have insisted on receiving, much more information about the new unit.

158

c. Dr. Ramsay and Dr. Dutton should have asked more questions about the way the unit was being run and taken suitable action if they were not satisfied with the replies. Lay people in management and administration should not have felt inhibited from questioning matters which they felt to be wrong simply because they were regarded as medical matters. (233–235).

Patient S

658. S was admitted to South Ockendon Hospital on 16 September 1969 after he had been convicted of indecent assault on an 8-year-old girl. (236–243)

659. Although S had no history of suicidal or violent tendencies and had never absconded from a hospital, he was kept in seclusion in a side room in the conditions described in paragraph 653 for 14 days after his admission and he remained in the security unit until 29 November. During this time his mother made vociferous and abusive complaints to the medical and nursing staff, to the Hospital Secretary, Dr. Dutton and Dr. Harfst without success. She then telephoned the Department of Health and Social Security who arranged for the RHB and HMC to investigate the complaints. Dr. Camm of the RHB visited the side room and wrote a sympathetic report on what he saw. Dr. Dutton then recommended that there should be an independent inquiry and the RHB invited Dr. Shapiro, Medical Superintendent of Harperbury Hospital, to visit and comment on the regime in Cypress Villa. (236 to 273).

660. We find that

a. every aspect of S's existence in the side room was unjustifiable.

b. the refusal of the nursing staff and of Dr. Benton to answer even simple questions led S's mother to become abusive.

c. the failure of Dr. Harfst to see S until 22 September was inexcusable, particularly in view of the complaints by the mother to him on 19 September.

d. Dr. Harfst's instructions on 22 September that S should remain longer in the side room were unjustified.

e. S would not have been let out of the side room by day on 30 September if it had not been for Dr. Camm's intervention.

f. although Dr. Dutton had heard from Dr. Ramsay of S's mother's complaint to the Department at least three days before, he was unable on 29 September to give Dr. Camm any explanation for the conditions in which S was being held. Whatever he felt to be the limitations of his powers of corrective action he should have made fuller enquiries than he did.

g. if Dr. Dutton was unhappy, as he claimed, about certain aspects of the regime in Cypress it was his duty as Physician Superintendent to let both the HMC and Dr. Ramsay know his views. He told neither.

h. if Dr. Shapiro had put in his letter of 13 October what he subsequently told Dr. Camm a month later it is unlikely that the HMC would have sanctioned Dr. Harfst's letter to S's mother warning her that she would not be allowed to visit if her behaviour did not improve.

i. the contemporary notes by Dr. Harfst and the nursing staff and Dr. Harfst's evidence about their dealings with S's mother revealed that

159

they were supporting each other in a hostile combination against her. Dr. Harfst should have been leading the staff away from retaliatory measures not lending them support.

j. but for the sustained campaign by S's mother he would not have been moved out of Cypress Villa in November 1969 or to another hospital in January 1970, and Cypress Villa would not have been closed as a security villa at that time. (291)

1969–1972: Cypress as a ward for disturbed patients

661. We find that when the use of Cypress Villa was changed from a security unit to a villa for disturbed patients Dr. Harfst took no steps to explain to the staff the effect of the change. In our opinion a clear policy should have been laid down and explained to the staff. (297 to 298)

John Meter

662. John Meter was transferred to Cypress Villa in December 1969 when he was 14 years old. He had presented a severe behaviour problem for many years, had proved ineducable and was liable to bite other patients and staff. Towards the end of 1971, John's behaviour deteriorated and he was reluctant to leave the side room, refused to wear clothes, refused to have furniture in the room, destroyed mattresses and fouled the floor and walls of his room (299 and 301).

663. Mrs. Meter, who visited her son frequently, complained that South Ockendon was not a suitable hospital for him and that the standard of care given in Cypress Villa caused his condition to deteriorate (304).

664. We find that
   a. South Ockendon Hospital was the only residential accommodation available and willing to take John Meter.
   b. the staff of South Ockendon Hospital are to be commended for their perseverance in caring for John and in seeking new ways to improve his condition.
   c. too little attention has been given to cleanliness, smell, heating and ventilation of the side room.
   d. the usual methods of drug and electrical treatment have been tried for John's condition, which is one for which there is as yet no known cure.
   e. the friction with Dr. Harfst in March 1972 was due to his inability to communicate in an understanding and friendly way with the concerned mother of a patient.
   f. the experiment in behaviour therapy was not persisted in long enough to judge whether it could prove valuable and the psychologist should have visited the ward to check on the progress being made before agreeing to the abandonment of the programme.
   g. the staff gave insufficient help to Mrs. Meter when she was willing to spend several hours a day at the hospital to help with the care of her son. It might still be possible to renew this potentially valuable experiment.
   h. a hospital for the mentally handicapped is at present more suitable than other places to care for John Meter. (323)

Allegations of violence in Cypress during 1972

665. We find that Mr. Dookhith lost his temper with *Patient U*, pulled him roughly from his chair and then kneed him. We are not able to say precisely where or with what force the knee made contact with U. We further find that while U was dragged through the day room he either fell or was pushed and that Mr. Dookhith kicked him two or three times in the region of the chest (330).

666. We find that the allegation that a blunt needle was used to give an injection to *patient PP* was without foundation. (332)

667. *Mrs. Meter* alleged that she saw a student nurse, Mr. Acero, holding a naked patient against the wall and punching him on the left ear. Mr. Acero replied that he was trying to prevent the patient from banging his face with his own hand. We find that Mr. Acero was using more force than was admitted or needed to control the patient, but we are not satisfied that he deliberately punched him on the ear. We think there was room for Mrs. Meter to have made an honest mistake as to what was happening. (333–335)

668. These episodes lead us to the view that too much force is not infrequently used to control violent or disobedient patients in Cypress Villa. (336)

Cypress Villa today

669. We find that there is still an excessive use of locked doors, that inadequate efforts are made to keep patients occupied and that the side rooms continue to be used for punishment purposes from time to time. Dr. Dutton, although claiming to have been unhappy about the regime, has done nothing about it because he regards it as being within the boundaries of Dr. Harfst's clinical autonomy. Dr. Harfst has failed to give adequate direction and guidance. The inadequate numbers of staff have done their best in most instances but lack proper guidance. (337–342)

Willows Villa

Allegations of Mrs. Youell

670. In December 1971, when Mrs. Youell began a spell of night duty, Willows Villa was the home of 48 subnormal and severely subnormal men. The consultant was Dr. Harfst. The nursing staff chiefly concerned were Miss Dooner, the unit nursing officer, Mr. Large and Mr. Turkington, day charge nurses, Mr. Macdonald, night superintendent, Mr. Margan, night charge nurse and Mrs. Youell, SEN. Mrs. Youell resigned on 17 February 1972 making the allegations set out in Appendix 7. The charge nurse against whom she made the allegation of lack of co-operation was Mr. Large (Chapter VI).

671. We find that Mrs. Youell was a very good and very conscientious nurse and that her standards were higher than those she found in Willows Ward. She suffered from anxiety which was aggravated by her inability to get the standard of care in Willows Ward improved. (352)

672. We find that Mr. Large wished to improve the conditions of the patients but easily became dissatisfied and discouraged when his attitude became surly. (353–356)

673. We deal with Mrs. Youell's allegations in paragraphs 674–704.

Patient C

674. Patient C, aged 75, had a chronic chest condition. He died on 6 February 1972.

675. We find that :
   a. when patient C became ill on the night of 30–31 January, Mr. Margan and Mr. Macdonald were at fault in not thinking it necessary to call a doctor to see him.
   b. when Dr. Motashaw saw C on 31 January she was in error in doubting the accuracy of Mrs. Youell's night report and deciding that there was nothing seriously wrong with him.
   c. the day staff failed to give proper nursing care to C on 31 January and Mr. Large was not justified in destroying the TPR chart started by Mrs. Youell.
   d. Mr. Macdonald should have sent for a doctor at 10.00 p.m. on 31 January. (362–363)

Patient D

676. We find that patient D fell on his way back from industrial therapy on 14 February 1972 and had skin lesions on both ankles. (364)

677. We find that Mr. Large should have made out an injury report and should have entered in the treatment book the Acetrin powder prescribed on 15 February by Dr. Benton. (365)

Patient E

678. Patient E, aged 63, who had been frail for some time died on 21 January. (366)

679. We find that when, on 18 January, E had a bad chest the day staff left it to the patient to decide whether to get up or stay in bed and gave no extra attention or small comforts to him. On 20 January he received insufficient fluids. (367–368)

Patient F

680. At about 6.30 p.m. on 31 January 1972 F fell over in the toilet area. He was assisted to bed and seen by Mr. Large who found no injury. Mrs. Youell, at Mr. Bartlett's request, looked at the leg before 9.00 p.m. and suspected a fracture. F then said he was not in pain but at 5.00 a.m. woke and said he had pain. He was seen at 5.30 a.m. by Dr. Benton and transferred to Gloucester Clinic where a fracture of the neck of the femur was diagnosed. (369)

681. We reject Mr. Large's evidence that he rotated both the patient's legs. We consider that he would have noticed the abnormal rotation of the leg if he had taken sufficient trouble and that he should have filled in an injury report and should have informed Mrs. Youell of the fall. (370)

682. We find that Mrs. Youell should have informed Mr. Margan or Mr. Macdonald of F's condition when they came to the villa, but that there were unusual circumstances which contributed to this failure. (370)

683. We find that Miss Dooner should have spoken to Mr. Large about his failure to make out an injury report or tell Mrs. Youell of F's fall. (370)

Patient H

684. Because of lack of evidence, we are unable to make a finding whether patient H was fit or unfit when he got up after a night-time seizure and an injection of paraldehyde. (371)

Patient J

685. J, aged 67, was seen by Mrs. Youell to be deteriorating during November and December 1971. He died on 5 April 1972. (372)

686. On the evidence before us we are not satisfied that J's health suffered as a result of his getting up on 31 January but he would have been more comfortable in bed. (373)

Patient K

687. K, aged 51, had a long history of skin disorders. Mrs. Youell believed that his leg was not being dressed as frequently as it should be and, in order to check this, marked a swab. (374)

688. We find that:
a. K did not receive proper care.
b. Mr. Large and Mr. Turkington failed
   i. to check that the dressings were being changed,
   ii. to see that the treatment and bath books were being properly kept. (375)

Patient Z

689. We find that when Mrs. Youell went on duty for the night of 14–15 February she found that there was no Gentian Violet, although this had been prescribed that day for patient Z about whom she had made a report on the previous night. (376)

Patient G

690. Patient G, aged 65, was unable to give a clear account of himself or of time and place. He had a mental age of less than seven years. He suffered from a speech defect and was very unsteady on his feet. He died on 13 February 1972. (379)

691. On the night of 10 February 1972 G vomited a large amount of bile. We find that Mr. Large should have asked a doctor to see G next day but that the vomit on this occasion was not connected with G's death. (379 and 380)

692. On the night of 12–13 February G vomited " coffee grounds " at 3.30 a.m. and there was projectile vomiting of green vomit at 5.30 a.m., when Mrs. Copland, the nurse on duty, noticed small bruises on his left eye and the bridge of his nose. On both occasions Mrs. Copland got in touch with Mr. Margan and he visited on the second occasion. He advised the giving of fluids and observation. We find that Mr. Margan should have gone to Willows Ward at 3.30 a.m. in

order to decide for himself whether he should call a doctor and that he was in error in not calling a doctor at 5.30 a.m. (379 and 380)

693. After breakfast on 14 February G again vomited "coffee grounds". At Dr. Benton's instigation, he was transferred to Gloucester Clinic at 10.30 a.m. At about midday G was found in a state of extreme shock and at 12.40 he produced a large amount of vomit and died. (379)

694. A post-mortem was carried out by Dr. Cameron who concluded that death was due to shock following severe bruising. It was suggested to the Coroner's jury on 2 May that the injuries could be explained by an incident which had occurred at the door leading from the day room to the toilet area at about 10.00 a.m. on 12 February. The jury returned a verdict of accidental death. (379 (vii) and 383)

695. We find that:
   a. a minor incident occurred in the doorway on 12 February when another patient pushed past G and caused him to fall to the floor. The incident was witnessed by 2 orderlies, Mr. Sharp and Mrs. Dawson, but Mr. Large and the other 2 nurses who were on duty said they did not see it. It is possible that injuries to the forehead, face and lip were caused at this time. (384–391)
   b. nothing occurred at that time which could account for the bruising of the abdomen and testicle. (391)
   c. we are unable to decide how G sustained the injuries to his abdomen, testicle and voice box. We are satisfied that no further investigation will solve this mystery. (392)

Re-education of patients
696. We find that Mrs. Youell on the one hand and Mr. Large and Mr. Turkington on the other hand held conflicting views on how best to educate patients not to hit other patients and that there was an unacceptable lack of policy or guidance on how the problems of misbehaviour by patients in Willows Ward should be dealt with. This was common to the whole hospital. (396)

Mrs. Youell's complaints of administrative deficiencies
697. We find that Mr. Large sometimes but not always went round the ward with Mrs. Youell when she took over from him. (397 (i))

698. We do not know whether Mr. Large read the nursing notes on which Mrs. Youell recorded information about patients not important enough for the ward report book but we are satisfied that he led Mrs. Youell to believe that he regarded them as a nuisance and of no value. (397 (ii))

699. We find that Mrs. Youell's complaint that patients kept buckets under their beds and urinated in them was justified. (397 (iii))

700. We find that Mrs. Youell was mistaken in wanting to have PRN drug lists and we accept the evidence of other witnesses that such lists should not be used. (397 (iv))

701. We find that an injection tray was not essential but its absence in Willows Ward was consistent with the low standards there. (397 (v))

702. We find the following further complaints to be true:—

a. the office cupboards were not labelled when Mrs. Youell started work in December. (397 (vi))

b. the patients' records were in a muddle and the X-ray forms difficult to find. (397 (vii))

c. the names of dead patients were still on the bedding list and on the beds. (397 (viii))

d. The day staff sometimes left the villa unswept with pools of urine on the floor. (397 (ix))

703. We accept that on occasions there was a flood in the toilets and they were dirty and we also accept Mr. Large's evidence that the pipes were too small and that the engineering staff had to clean them frequently. (397 (x))

704. We find that Mr. Large told Mrs. Youell in December 1971 that he had got rid of a previous night nurse because he was always finding bruises and scratches on patients and making out accident reports and we believe that this assertion was probably correct. (404)

Allegations of Mrs. Woods

705. Mrs. Woods, a former pupil nurse at South Ockendon Hospital, made allegations of unkindness to patients in Willows Ward by Mr. Auchoybur, a pupil nurse, and Mrs. Balah, a nursing assistant, on various occasions in February 1972.

706. We accept Mrs. Woods' evidence, which was supported by notes she had written at the time and we find that:

a. Mr. Auchoybur tripped up two patients on separate occasions.

b. Mr. Auchoybur and Mrs. Balah teased another patient by taking away his handkerchief and throwing it backwards and forwards to each other; and that on another occasion Mr. Auchoybur hit this patient on the head with a rag doll causing the patient to retaliate by picking up a chair to hit Mr. Auchoybur.

c. incidents as in a. and b. were regarded as a joke among the nursing staff generally including at least one charge nurse. Had the charge nurses been doing their job properly, the incidents would not have occurred.

d. on 12 February Mrs. Balah handled patient G roughly when hurrying him to his bath and caused him to fall backwards into the bath. We are satisfied that he suffered no injury as a result of this. (417–420)

General standard of care in December 1971 to February 1972 and its causes

707. We find that the care of patients in Willows Ward during this period seldom exceeded the bare minimum and often fell below it. Examples of the low standard of care are given in earlier paragraphs, for example paragraphs 679, 689, 699.

708. We find that *Mr. Margan*, the night charge nurse, though he had previously had a high regard for Mrs. Youell as a nurse and found her cheerful and uncomplaining made no attempt to find out the cause of her dissatisfaction with standards in Willows Ward during this period. He regarded her complaints as

165

trivial, was annoyed by her complaining attitude and was anxious to have as little to do with her as possible. (400–402)

709. We find that *Mr. Macdonald*, the night superintendent, also regarded the complaints as trivial and they were all settled to his satisfaction by his speaking to Mr. Large and Miss Dooner. He agreed that Mr. Large never disputed the validity of any complaint. (403)

710. We find that *Miss Dooner*, the unit nursing officer, was not able to exercise sufficient supervision of Willows Villa and that Mr. Large and Mr. Turkington did not pay much attention to her unless it suited them. (405–406)

711. We find that *Mr. Hubbard*, the senior nursing officer, left it to the discretion of the unit nursing officers how often to check records, how to carry out their supervisory duties and what information to feed back to him about nursing standards in the villas. (408–410)

712. We find that criticism from those below was resented or ignored wherever possible and there was a reluctance to give any subordinate any clear directions. (411)

713. We find that the attitudes and capabilities of the nursing staff described in paragraphs 708–711 reveal why the nursing administration failed to detect or halt the declining standards in Willows Ward. (411–412)

714. We find that the medical care was on occasions below that which we would have expected to find. (416)

Result of complaining

715. We find that Mrs. Youell was ostracised by many of the staff after making her allegations and resigning. (421 (ii))

716. We find that Mrs. Woods did not report the incidents of unkindness which she saw to her senior officers in the hospital for fear of losing her job. (417 (vi), 421 (ii))

Willows Villa today

717. We find that both the accommodation and the provision for occupation has been improved but in this as in some other villas the best use is not being made of the time of the nursing staff. (422)

Other Villas

718. The great majority of letters received, mainly from the relatives of patients and former patients, praised very highly the care given by the staff, despite overcrowding and understaffing. (425–431)

719. We find that the standard of care varies widely. It is high in some villas but tends to be least satisfactory in the villas for severely subnormal and disturbed men and boys. The quality of the staff of each villa is the dominating factor in determining the standard of care but all villas are affected by shortage of trained staff and most villas by overcrowding and other weaknesses in the accommodation. Gloucester Clinic, the medical centre, maintains a very high standard and the management of the new houses at Gloucester Drive has made a good start. (432–446)

Occupation and Recreation

720. We find that the present accommodation and staff available for occupational and industrial therapy are inadequate and more of both is needed. (452–455, 460–464 and 478–479)

721. We find that recreational activities are varied and enterprising and some excellent schemes are being organised on individual wards by charge nurses as well as centrally by the Recreations Officer. Many of the nursing staff give their own time to help with these activities. (465–471 and 476–477)

722. We consider that the hospital is fortunate to have a large number of voluntary helpers, including schoolchildren, who take a keen and practical interest in the patients and have been instrumental in making their lives happier. (472–475)

General Matters

The Regional Hospital Board

723. We find that the Regional Hospital Board :
   a. should have realised the danger of overcrowding and understaffing earlier than it did and should have taken action earlier instead of pinning undue hopes on the relief to be given by local authority hostels. (32, 141–142, 491)
   b. should have laid down a policy for Cypress Villa and taken steps to see whether it was functioning satisfactorily. (180–181, 490)
   c. should have shown better judgment when appointing a Chairman to the Hospital Management Committee in 1969. (491 and 522)
   d. should have made sure that a workable multi-disciplinary structure was in operation at the hospital after Dr. Dutton ceased to be Physician Superintendent in 1972. (491, 506–507)

The Hospital Management Committee

724. We find that the Hospital Management Committee :
   a. have taken too restricted a view of their duty towards the patients, have left policy and management in the hands of the consultants and have wrongly regarded the way of life in each villa as lying within the clinical autonomy of the consultant.
   b. have failed to give proper consideration to matters of policy such as those raised by the report of the Hospital Advisory Service.
   c. have concentrated on matters of detail which should have been dealt with by officers.
   d. have insisted on retaining an inefficient and time-wasting committee structure against the advice of Department of Health and Social Security and the Hospital Advisory Service.
   e. have not been sufficiently concerned with good staff relationships. (494–521)

Medical staff and standard of medical care

725. We find that *Dr. Dutton's* ideas have been sound but he has lacked the drive necessary to translate his ideas into a working policy and to see that it was

implemented. His laissez-faire approach and over-high regard for the clinical autonomy of other consultants contributed to the continuance of the unjustifiable regime in Cypress Villa. (524–527, 232 (iv), 291 (vii) and 342).

726. We find than *Dr. Harfst* needed more support and guidance in his first consultant post than he either asked for or received. The regime which he introduced in Cypress Villa was insensitive and inhumane and his handling of the complaints flowing from it was inept. We believe that many of his mistakes stemmed from his own lack of security and that he has learnt from them. We consider that he is now far more able to do the job required of him at South Ockendon than he was when he was appointed and that working within a team he will succeed. (528 and Chapter V)

727. We find that the standard of medical care in Gloucester Clinic was very high, but the patients who were nursed in their villas received a more variable standard. In Willows Villa the medical supervision failed to lift the unacceptably low nursing standard. (529)

Nursing staff and standard of nursing care

728. We find that the Chief Nursing Officer and Principal Nursing Officer are making changes for the better. (537)

729. We find that some of the nurses in middle management are not of adequate calibre. (537)

730. We find that the charge nurses are of varying capabilities but that a considerable number of them are able and enthusiastic. Others need greater supervision by and encouragement from their unit nursing officers. (538)

731. We find that the best use is not being made of the limited nursing resources. (545)

732. We find that the employment of nurses with an inadequate command of the English language is most unsatisfactory. (543)

Lay administration

733. We find that the sub-committee structure of the Hospital Management Committee and the attention of all committees to matters of detail have made it impossible for the Group Secretary and his colleagues to do their job as it should be done. (556)

The handling of complaints

734. We are satisfied that it needs a great deal of courage for a member of the staff to comment on the way an individual carries out his or her work and that people who have shown that courage have too often had occasion to regret it. (558–574 and 421 (ii))

735. We find that criticism by parents or relatives is resented by many of the staff and that complaints by patients are often ignored. (560–569, 577)

736. We find that there is a tendency to give undue support to people who have been the subject of criticism. (575–576)

Catering

737. We find that the catering generally gives satisfaction but we agree with the view of the hospital authorities in their evidence that there is room for improvement. (578, 583)

Laundry

738. We find that the inadequacy of the laundry, of which the hospital authorities are aware, is one of the reasons why patients are not yet able to have personal clothing. (584-585)

Contribution of Local Authorities

739. We find Local Authorities are unable to accept into the community patients from South Ockendon Hospital whom they acknowledge to be suitable for community care. This is because of inadequate provision of residential homes. The existence of these patients in hospital prevents the admission of others who are in need of hospital care. (588–591 and 597)

Reduction of overcrowding

740. We find that the hospital is now near to achieving the interim target of a minimum of 50 square feet of bed space and 30 square feet of day space for each patient and a maximum of 50 patients in adult wards and 30 patients in children's wards. (595–596)

Recommendations

Multi-disciplinary Control

1. There should be multi-disciplinary determination and control of the standard of care to be achieved throughout the hospital. Our report suggests a possible framework consisting of formal multi-disciplinary teams at hospital and unit level and less formal multi-disciplinary contacts in each villa together with an Activities Team concerned with all forms of occupation and recreation in the hospital.

2. The individual responsibility of consultants towards their patients in strictly clinical matters should not be allowed to conflict with policy decisions of the hospital multi-disciplinary team on general principles of care in the villas or to impede the work of the unit multi-disciplinary teams.

3. The hospital multi-disciplinary team should translate guidance from the Department, Board and Group into a working policy and see that it is carried out in the villas. This will include general guidance on such matters as the proper use of side rooms and the locking of doors, and ensuring that the best use is made of the existing resources.

4. Adequate secretarial and clerical assistance should be provided for the multi-disciplinary teams.

5. The allocation of villas to consultants and unit nursing officers should be adjusted so that, as far as possible, the villas under a unit nursing officer are the responsibility of one consultant.

169

Management

6. The committee structure of the Hospital Management Committee should be reorganised on the lines recommended in HM(68)28.

7. The Group Secretary, with the co-operation of the Chairman of the Medical Executive Committee, the Chief Nursing Officer and other professional officers should ensure that matters of policy are brought before the Hospital Management Committee with prior circulation of papers setting out the facts and arguments and a clear indication of the matters requiring policy decisions.

8. The Hospital Management Committee should concentrate on matters of principle and policy and should, wherever possible, frame their decisions in such a way as to permit delegation to officers of the detailed implementation of the principles the Hospital Management Committee have laid down.

9. The Hospital Management Committee should have a written policy for dealing with and reporting acts of violent behaviour and should ensure that all staff receive a copy of it.

Handling of Complaints

10. Nursing staff should be helped to understand the concern of parents of mentally handicapped patients and not to resent their criticism.

11. Members of staff to whom a complaint is made by a patient should report it in writing to the charge nurse (or other appropriate senior officer). The charge nurse should transmit the complaint to the consultant and unit officer for action in the light of the complaints procedures currently in force.

12. Whenever a charge of negligence is made against staff, the acts or omissions upon which the charge is based should be clearly set out.

Standards of Care

Medical staff

13. Where the Chairman of the Medical Executive Committee becomes aware of problems within the clinical responsibility of a consultant he should discuss them with the consultant and if no satisfactory solution can be achieved should report the matter to the Senior Administrative Medical Officer.

Nursing staff

14. Action should be taken to improve the standard of leadership and supervision in middle management.

15. Particular attention should be given by senior nursing officers and nursing officers to villas with special problems.

16. Where guidance is needed, clear directions should be given to subordinates.

17. Criticism and comment from junior nurses should be considered and followed by investigation where necessary. It should not be ignored or resented.

18. The nursing establishment should be revised to take account of the reduction of the working week from 42 to 40 hours.

19. It would be an advantage if one of the two charge nurses normally working in a villa could be given overall responsibility for the villa.

20. The extent of the hospital's dependence on staff with an inadequate knowledge of English should be made known to those concerned with determining the remuneration and conditions of service of nurses.

21. Further consideration should be given to the possibility of extending the London Weighting to this hospital.

22. There should be a full-time nursing officer to organise in-service training of nursing staff.

23. The standard of care should not admit indignities such as a queue of naked patients for baths and infrequent shaving.

24. The slapping of patients should never be permitted.

Accommodation

25. Urgent measures should be taken to reach in every villa the minimum standard of 30 square feet day space and 50 square feet bed space per patient and to reduce the numbers of patients in adult wards below 50 and in children's wards below 30.

26. The numbers of patients in Beech and Poplars Villas should be reduced to 30 by the end of 1973.

27. More accommodation should be provided for Occupational and Industrial Therapy.

28. Arrangements should be made for the use or provision of indoor accommodation for vigorous games.

29. WCs in villas should be screened from corridors.

30. The need for further staff accommodation should be assessed.

Occupation

31. Pending the provision of more accommodation for the occupation of patients, the number of nursing staff allocated to occupying patients on the wards should be increased.

32. The Activities Team mentioned in Recommendation 1 should organise the best use of the staff and other resources available for occupying patients in various ways.

General

33. Central guidance should be issued to hospital authorities on the operation of the Cogwheel medical structure, the Salmon Nursing structure and multi-disciplinary teams in a hospital for mentally handicapped patients.

Cypress Villa

34. The following alterations should be made to the side rooms:
    a. The handle and lock of the door should be altered to permit opening from the inside when the door is not locked.
    b. The ventilation and, when necessary, the heating should be improved.

35. As many nurses as is reasonably possible should be allocated to the care of disturbed patients like John Meter and they should be cared for in smaller groups.

1974

36. When the proposed new Community Health Council for the area is created, some people should be appointed because of their existing interest and work in South Ockendon Hospital.

J. HAMPDEN INSKIP
HARRY MCCREE
PATIENCE SHEARD
ERIC W. SHEPHERD
JOHN WILLS

EVIDENCE RECEIVED BY THE COMMITTEE

A. Persons who gave Written and Oral Evidence

North-East Metropolitan Regional Hospital Board
Sir Graham Rowlandson—Chairman.
Mr. R. Huws Jones—Former Member.
Mr. L. C. Phipps—Secretary.
Professor T. A. Ramsay—Former Senior Administrative Medical Officer.
Dr. P. M. C. Camm—Principal Assistant Senior Medical Officer.

South Ockendon Group Hospital Management Committee
Mr. W. A. Nichols—Chairman.
Mr. G. S. Whiting—Vice-Chairman.
Mr. G. W. Hood—Former Member.
Mr. M. N. Harrison—Group Secretary.

Hospital Staff
Mr. H. G. Alger—State Enrolled Nurse.
Mr. J. M. Andrews—Chief Nursing Officer.
Mrs. A. G. Balah—Nursing Assistant.
Mr. J. A. Bass—Ward Orderly.
Mr. C. E. Beacham—Student Nurse.
Dr. M. D. Benton—Medical Assistant.
Mr. D. A. Blackburn—Clinical Psychologist.
Mr. G. Campanella—Charge Nurse.
Mr. M. Charnier—Student Nurse.
Mrs. I. Chatting—Ward Orderly.
Mr. D. Crowson—Charge Nurse.
Mr. W. Davies—Nursing Officer.
Mrs. V. A. Dawson—Ward Orderly.
Mr. A. F. Dookhith—Pupil Nurse.
Miss M. B. Dooner—Nursing Officer.
Dr. G. Dutton—Chairman, Medical Executive Committee; Consultant Psychiatrist.
Mr. R. A. Essop—Pupil Nurse.
Miss M. S. Gibberd—Occupational Therapist.
Mr. A. Hardas—Charge Nurse.
Dr. M. J. Harfst—Consultant Psychiatrist.
Mr. J. J. Heffernan—Principal Nursing Officer.
Mr. R. B. Hubbard—Senior Nursing Officer.
Mr. N. Jairam—Pupil Nurse.
Mr. A. T. Knopp—State Enrolled Nurse.
Mr. P. Laide—Senior Nursing Officer.
Mr. C. G. Lewis—Nursing Officer.

Mrs. M. A. R. Linnegar—Nursing Assistant.
Mr. A. Macdonald—Night Superintendent.
Mr. A. A. Maghoo—State Enrolled Nurse.
Mr. D. Margan—Night Charge Nurse.
Mr. K. K. Mitra—Staff Nurse.
Mrs. C. O'Brien—Nursing Assistant.
Mr. M. J. Prentis—Nursing Assistant.
Mrs. R. Samson—Nursing Assistant.
Mr. D. J. Schreeche-Powell—Charge Nurse.
Mr. W. R. Searle—Senior Nursing Officer.
Mr. J. C. Shrimpton—Senior State Enrolled Nurse.
Mr. F. G. Smith—Charge Nurse.
Mr. D. Taylor—Ward Orderly.
Mr. F. D. Toal—Charge Nurse.
Mr. R. W. Turkington—Charge Nurse.
Mr. P. J. Walsh—Night Charge Nurse.
Mr. G. F. Wood—Nursing Officer.
Dr. M. E. York-Moore—Consultant Psychiatrist.
Mr. H. L. Yu—Pupil Nurse.

Former Hospital Staff*

Mr. L. Balsdon—Staff Nurse.
Mr. W. G. Bartlett—Nursing Assistant.
Mr. A. M. Emambocus—State Enrolled Nurse.
Mr. A. Findlay—Charge Nurse.
Mr. J. F. Hunnam—Pupil Nurse.
Dr. D. C. Jones—Medical Assistant.
Dr. M. Kant—Registrar.
Mr. D. R. Large—Charge Nurse.
Mr. R. Moothoo—Student Nurse.
Dr. Motashaw—General Practitioner (deceased).
Mr. J. A. Powell—Student Nurse.
Mr. C. A. Sharp—Ward Orderly.
Mr. P. S. Willingham—Charge Nurse.
Mrs. D. J. Woods—Pupil Nurse.
Mrs. M. R. Youell—State Enrolled Nurse.

Others

Mr. H. G. Atkins—Father of a former patient.
Dr. G. Bram—Consultant Psychiatrist.
Mr. S. A. Brand—Detective Constable.
Dr. J. M. Cameron—Pathologist.
Brother of Patient S.
Mr. R. Eason—Detective Sergeant.
Mother of Patients PP and NN.
Mother of Patient T.
Father of Patient V.
Mr. R. Hill—Labourer.

*Grades given are those applying before departure from the hospital.

Mr. D. T. Lynch—Police Constable.
Mrs. G. J. McWilliams—Niece of a patient.
Mrs. M. Meter—Mother of a patient.
Chief Superintendent A. R. Mitchell.
Mr. R. A. Nelson—Carpenter.
Mr. F. J. Pryor—Chairman, League of Friends.
Mrs. P. Read—Mother of a former patient.
Mrs. C. Smart—Mother of a former patient.
Dr. G. Stores—Consultant Psychiatrist.
Dr. D. C. Taylor—Consultant Psychiatrist.
Mrs. I. A. Thorne—Member, League of Friends.
Dr. J. P. Whitehead—Pathologist.

B. Persons who gave Oral Evidence only

Hospital Staff

Mr. E. Acero—Nursing Assistant.
Mrs. K. Archer—Nursing Officer.
Mr. A. S. Auchoybur—Pupil Nurse.
Mrs. N. Bartlett—Ward Sister.
Mr. G. C. Bird—Charge Nurse.
Mrs. E. A. Bugg—Nursing Officer.
Mr. R. E. D. Champion—Charge Nurse.
Mrs. A. M. Copland—Nursing Assistant.
Mr. I. Fokheer—Pupil Nurse.
Mrs. C. Greig—Nursing Assistant.
Mr. K. Harding—Charge Nurse.
Miss E. Hutterer—Headmistress.
Mr. W. Kellock—Consultant Surgeon.
Mr. A. T. Lewis—Officer in Charge of Industrial Therapy.
Mrs. M. L. McLay—Nursing Officer.
Mrs. J. Peggs—Ward Sister.
Mr. A. R. Romjon—State Enrolled Nurse.
Mr. A. M. Schreeche-Powell—Charge Nurse.

Former Hospital Staff*

Mr. G. McFadyen—Charge Nurse.

Others

Mrs. D. C. Bird—Mother of a patient.
Mr. T. E. N. Driberg—Member of Parliament.
Detective Superintendent G. A. Harris.
Patient KK.
Mr. J. E. Morris—Treasury Solicitor's Department.
Dr. A. Shapiro—Consultant Psychiatrist.
Father of Patient TT.

---

*Grades given are those applying before departure from the hospital.

C. Persons who submitted Written Evidence only

Department of Health and Social Security

Mr. W. F. Farrant—Assistant Secretary.

North-East Metropolitan Regional Hospital Board

Mr. G. H. Clarke—Treasurer.
Miss S. G. White—Regional Nursing Officer.

Hospital Management Committee (Members)

Mr. S. G. Crabb.
Dr. J. A. C. Franklin.
Mr. G. F. Howard.
Mr. T. R. Newman.
Mrs. O'Shea.
Mrs. Protheroe.
Mrs. F. E. Watson.
Mrs. A. V. Winch.

Hospital Staff

Mrs. A. Alder—Nursing Assistant.
Mrs. E. Barlow—Domestic Supervisor.
Mrs. J. G. Jarman—Nursing Assistant.
Mrs. D. Mobsby—State Enrolled Nurse.
Mr. C. B. Offord—Hospital Secretary.
Mr. J. I. Purdie—Tutor.
Mr. P. B. Tester—Nursing Officer.
Mr. G. L. Thomas—Voluntary Services Organiser.
Mrs. B. Thompson—Ward Sister.

Former Staff*

Mr. W. J. Blevins—Tutor.
Mrs. D. Keeling—Nursing Assistant.
Dr. S. Leeks—Registrar.
Mrs. I. Milbourn—Nursing Assistant.
Mr. A. M. Pegley—Deputy Chief Male Nurse.
Mrs. G. A. Tollinton—Senior Clinical Psychologist.

Others

Patient D.
Mrs. Comber—Mother of a patient.
Patient S.
Dr. C. Finn—Consultant Psychiatrist.
Mr. P. Ginever—Church of Scientology.
Mrs. S. Greenblatt—Mother of a patient.
Mr. J. Kukulak—Friend of a patient.
Mr. and Mrs. S. J. Lane—Parents of a patient.

*Grades given are those applying before departure from the hospital.

Mrs. J. Neild—Mother of a former patient.
Mrs. B. Robb—Chairman, Aid for the Elderly in Government Institutions.
Mrs. E. Reeves—Mother of a patient.
Mr. D. R. Sansom—Father of a patient.
Mr. J. T. Smith—Father of a patient.
Mr. L. Woolley—Father of a patient.

APPENDIX 2

PARTIES AND LEGAL REPRESENTATIVES

Party	Legal Representatives
Committee of Inquiry	Mr. J. A. C. Spokes, Barrister-at-Law and Mr. M. J. L. Brodrick, Barrister-at-Law, instructed by the Treasury Solicitor.
North-East Metropolitan Regional Hospital Board	Mr. D. Latham, Barrister-at-Law and Mr. R. Bell, Barrister-at-Law, instructed by Mr. T. R. Dibley, Legal Adviser to the Regional Hospital Board.
South Ockendon Hospital Group Hospital Management Committee	Mr. R. Croxon, Barrister-at-Law instructed by Hatton, Jewers and Mepham, Basildon, Essex.
Mr. M. Harrison ... ... Mr. C. Offord	Mr. C. Smith, Barrister-at-Law instructed by Mr. J. G. Haley, Solicitor, National and Local Government Officers Association.
Dr. G. Dutton ... ... Dr. M. Benton Dr. M. York-Moore Dr. J. Hurst	Mr. A. Brooks, Barrister-at-Law, instructed by Hempson and Co., Henrietta Street, London.
Dr. M. J. Harfst	Mr. G. Bovell, Solicitor, of Le Brasseur and Oakley, Great Russell Street, London.
Dr. D. C. Jones	Mr. R. Sumerling, Solicitor, of Le Brasseur and Oakley, Great Russell Street, London.
Mr. J. M. Andrews ... ... Mr. W. R. Searle Mr. R. B. Hubbard	Mr. T. Walker, Barrister-at-Law, instructed by Charles Russell and Co., Lincoln's Inn, London.
Mr. D. R. Large	Mr. C. Nicolls, Barrister-at-Law, instructed by Hewitt and Co., Dartford, Kent.
Mr. J. H. Powell	Mr. M. Selfe, Barrister-at-Law, instructed by Talbot, Copner and Davies, Andover, Hampshire.
Members of the Confederation of Health Service Employees	Mr. E. A. G. Spanswick, Assistant General Secretary of Confederation of Health Service Employees.

178

STAFF AND BEDS, NUMBERS AND RATIOS

Table A

Medical staff—South Ockendon Sub-group*

	Available Staffed Beds at 30 December	||Patients in South Ockendon Sub-Group	Number of consultants at 30 September	Ratio of consultants to patients		Number of other medical staff at 30 September	Ratio of other medical staff to patients		Total Medical Staff at 30 September	Ratio of patients to medical staff	
				South Ockendon Sub-Group	†National		South Ockendon Sub-Group	†National		South Ockendon Sub-Group	†National
1966	1228·9	1163	2 1/11	1:556·2	1:513·2	4	1:290·63	1:365·2	6 1/11	1:190·9	1:213·4
1968	1248	1165	3 2/11	1:363·2	1:521·4	4	1:291	1:346·6	7 2/11	1:165·1	1:208·2
1969	1239	1137	3 6/11	1:320·7	1:443·5	4	1:284·2	1:343·9	7 6/11	1:150·6	1:193·7
1970	1180	1117	3 4/11	1:331·8	1:442·1	3	1:372	1:331·8	6 4/11	1:175·3	1:189·6
1971	1155	1061	3 9/11	1:277·8	1:407·5	2 9/11	1:376·5	1:311·1	6 7/11	1:159·8	1:176·4

\|\|Average Daily Bed Occupancy.

*Figures relate to South Ockendon Hospital, Little Warley Lodge, New Lodge Hospital, Duvals Hostel and Ramsey Lodge Hospital.

†England and Wales.

STAFF AND BEDS, NUMBERS AND RATIOS

APPENDIX 3

Nursing staff—South Ockendon Hospital

Table B

| | Available staffed beds as at 30 December | §Patients | Number of qualified* nursing staff at 30 September | Ratio of qualified nursing staff to patients | | Number of unqualified nursing staff at 30 September | Ratio of unqualified nursing staff to patients | | Total number of nursing staff at 30 September | Ratio of nursing staff to patients | |
				South Ockendon Hospital	†National		South Ockendon Hospital	‡National		South Ockendon Hospital	†National
1966	1045·9	982·4	73·1	1:13·44	1:11·9	175·4	1:5·60	1:6·8	276·2	1:3·55	1:4·3
1968	1065	988	142·1‖	1:6·95	1:6·5	133·5	1:7·40	1:10·4	275·6	1:3·58	1:4·00
1969	1052	958	151·6	1:6·32	1:6·7	124·2	1:7·71	1:9·1	275·8	1:3·47	1:3·9
1970	980	922	165·7	1:5·56	1:6·2	125·8	1:7·33	1:8·00	291·5	1:3·16	1:3·5
1971	955	866	169·9	1:5·34	1:6·0	160·1	1:5·41	1:6·4	330	1:2·47	1:3·1
1972	945	†	162·0	†	†	217·7	†	†	379·7	†	†

§Average Daily Bed Occupancy.

*Qualified includes administrative staff.

‖From 1968 the qualified figure includes State Enrolled Nurses who up to that year were counted as unqualified.

†England and Wales

‡Information not available.

Census of Mentally Handicapped Patients in Hospital in England and Wales 1970
Mentally Handicapped Patients with Severe Incapacities and Behaviour Problems
Numbers and Percentages[1]

Incapacities and behaviour problems	Hospitals and units for mentally handicapped. England and Wales			South Ockendon Hospital		
	All	Degree of Mental Handicap		All	Degree of Mental Handicap	
		Severe	Mild		Severe	Mild
	Numbers					
Total population	56,958	40,899	16,059	912	705	207
Non-ambulant	7,359	6,525	834	168	141	27
Severe behaviour difficulty	8,769	7,362	1,407	156	144	12
Severely incontinent	11,901	11,244	657	258	240	18
Needs much help to feed, wash and dress ...	13,509	12,879	630	291	276	15
	Per cent					
Non-ambulant	12·9	16·0	5·2	18·4	20·0	13·0
Severe behaviour difficulty	15·4	18·0	8·8	17·1	20·4	5·8
Severely incontinent	20·9	27·5	4·1	28·3	34·0	8·7
Needs much help to feed, wash and dress ...	23·7	31·5	3·9	31·9	39·3	7·3

[1] Patients counted more than once.

Mr. Harrison
Secretary
South Ockendon Group Hospital
  Management Committee
Leytonstone House
High Road
LONDON E11   *13 January 1969*

Dear Mr. Harrison

PATIENT OVERCROWDING IN THE SOUTH OCKENDON GROUP

The above subject was discussed at a recent meeting of the Group Medical Advisory Committee. The Physician Superintendent, supported fully by his colleagues, reported to that committee on evils attendant upon this state of affairs which exists in the group at the present time. The views which he expressed were strongly endorsed by all members of the committee present, and it was agreed that it should be made known to the Hospital Management Committee what the true situation is with regard to patient overcrowding in the group, what effects it has and why it is that those who are immediately concerned with patient care look upon it with such grave concern. I therefore report to you as follows:

I refer firstly to a memorandum issued by the last Group Secretary and dated 1 July 1961. In that memorandum it is made clear that overcrowding had occurred in South Ockendon Hospital as judged by inpatient bed numbers over and above the original recommended statutory beddages of the then existing wards. It would appear from the figures quoted that the official overall degree of overcrowding was believed to be in the region of 15 per cent. The memorandum goes on to state that the Hospital Management Committee has agreed and the Regional Board has concurred in the revision of authorised accommodation in the hospital to a new set of figures, that is those representing the 15 per cent degree of overcrowding.

I refer secondly to the latest Regional Board Handbook of information on hospital services, dated August 1966. It quotes these sets of figures (which I reproduce for you at the end of this letter) which indicate that the degree of patient overcrowding everywhere in the hospital group as measured by numbers of beds being used over and above accommodation receiving recognised staffed standards is very considerably more than 15 per cent. The overall average degree of overcrowding calculated from these figures is in the region of 47 per cent. The degree of overcrowding in South Ockendon Hospital, Leytonstone House and Great West Hatch, Chigwell, approach this figure whilst the degree of overcrowding at Ramsay Lodge is 55 per cent, that at New Lodge 57 per cent, and that at Little Warley Lodge no less than 79 per cent.

The latest building regulations of 1964 recommend for hospital beds for **our** type of patient a minimum distance of 7 ft between the centres of adjacent **beds.**

I have not discovered in South Ockendon Hospital any ward where this figure appertains, except the Gloucester Clinic which, because of its special function, conforms to General Hospital standards, and Cypress Villa. It does not even hold for the new Laurels Villa, which contains more children within one unit than modern planners would recommend. This means that by all reasonable standards there is overcrowding of patients in South Ockendon Hospital and worse in other parts of the group.

The effect of this overcrowding on living standards must not be underestimated. It means that privacy is virtually impossible for patients. It means that most patients cannot have any control over their private property or keep anything safely within convenient distance of their beds, since there is no room for individual bedside lockers. Indeed nothing but the barest minimum of private property can be stored at all in the wards. It must be remembered that very many patients spend their lives in these wards and have to try and structure their entire existence round these unsatisfactory living conditions. Part of our job is to try and train them in the skills of acquiring and keeping private property, in spending their wages, etc., earned in other departments of the hospital.

Overcrowding is not, of course, simply a matter of space between beds and space for storage of private property. Day room accommodation and airing court space is similarly grossly inadequate in many wards. This is particularly so in children's wards and those housing severely subnormal refractory patients. There is a lack of partitioning and smaller day room and side room accommodation, leading to the situation where large numbers of disturbed patients are held together in one room. Gross degradation of human behaviour follows amongst low-grade patients living under these conditions. The more disturbed members of such a community cause further disturbance in the rest, leading to increasingly uncontrollable behaviour in the whole group. In the case of refractory patients, the incidence of violence increases, and perusal of the daily returns of reports of injury to ward staff gives a measure of the size of the problem which has to be tackled at the present time. To give an example of how the patient load has outstripped facilities, the case of Beeches Ward at South Ockendon can be quoted. This ward contains 52 severely subnormal refractory male patients, about half of whom are periodically violent. A nucleus of about a dozen of them are regularly and recurrently violent, and this violence occasionally reaches homicidal proportions. The ward has one side room only to deal with these patients. It is in almost constant use, and often patients have to take turns to enter it. Patients have to be removed from it before they are ready to accommodate someone in even greater need. Quite often violent patients have to be isolated in a lobby in the lavatory, and this used as a temporary side room. Fortunately the situation on Beeches Villa is about to be relieved to some extent by the timely provision of some further side rooms.

Overcrowding appears to us to be the key factor in a viciously spiralling process of falling standards of patient care. It is an affront to human dignity when, as is often the case, one patient has to wait for colleagues sleeping adjacent to enter their beds before he can get into his own, and when children supposedly cot-bound can travel down the length of the dormitory, progressing from cot to cot by climbing over the short space between them.

Sanitary standards deteriorate as a result of patient overcrowding, and in the type of patient with which we deal many rapidly reach a critical phase threatening the community health of the whole hospital. There is a high rate of staphylococeal skin infections among patients, resulting in persistent and recurrent boils, carbuncles and skin rashes. This involves much medical and nursing time, patient discomfort and expense on account of the use of the costly antibiotics required in treatment. Staphylococeal infections, moreover, are potentially serious. Whipworm infestation has been introduced into the community and has spread rapidly. Its management and eradication are matters of great difficulty and again involve much time and expense. Scabies infestation is now virtually endemic in South Ockendon Hospital. A recent outbreak involved every patient in one ward and nearly all the staff. This is a highly infectious condition, most distressing and uncomfortable to experience, and management and treatment are again costly and time consuming.

The nursing staff are asked to continue their work in this deteriorating situation. Inadequate in numbers to deal with this vast patient load and unable to make any significant impression upon the problems created by these large numbers, they are forced to stand by, frustrated and helpless, mindful of what could be done under different circumstances. Job dissatisfaction is a thing we could well do without under our present difficulties.

Recent experiments in the field of social psychiatry have indicated that significant achievements can be brought about in the care of disturbed and mentally retarded patients in terms of improved behaviour, increased socialisation, rise in functioning intellectual ability, educability and response to training programmes, if they are nursed and trained in an environment in which overcrowding is reduced, that is if they are in relatively small groups with adequate living space and a high staff-patient ratio. These conditions do not exist in the group at the present time.

It is not known what potential our patients may have for further training and education. It is certainly appreciable and may be crucial. As an investment such programmes are likely to result in rehabilitation, discharge and resettlement for some patients. All patients have a right to have their talents and abilities exercised to the full. The responsibility for seeing that this is done and that each individual patient's potential is realised as completely as possible rests with us who are in charge of their care. We believe that no training programme can succeed in the long term if the present degree of overcrowding is allowed to continue, nor can we compete successfully with other hospital groups or other specialties in terms of standards of patient care.

We believe that the reduction of overcrowding in the hospital group is a matter of great urgency. It is also, of course, a matter of great difficulty while pressure for admission of further urgent cases in the community is so great and the discharge rate is so low. Nevertheless we search for every conceivable means to bring it about.

We hope that you will bear these points in mind in your future deliberations on this subject and that the Management Committee will continue to do everything within its power in its negotiations with the Regional Board to secure substantial reductions in our inpatient complement.

Yours sincerely
M. J. HARFST
Honorary Secretary
South Ockendon Group
Medical Advisory Committee

SOUTH OCKENDON HOSPITAL

14 April 1972

Re: John Meter

This young man has been in a state of equilibrium for many months now, if we can accept that the refusal to wear clothes, to use a bed or bedding, to destroy every mattress given to him within two or three days, to urinate on the floor, to defaecate and smear faeces over himself and the walls of his room, to refuse to leave his room, and to insist that the door of his room is locked and that he is left alone.

If these situations do not pertain, then John becomes disturbed. He bites, pinches, will grab at the Male Nurses' testes, breaks windows with his head, pushes any furniture out of any room in which he may find himself.

John cannot tolerate the presence of any other person and will scream most piercingly and kick the door or wall with his bare foot if people remain anywhere near him. If left or taken into the presence of other patients he will immediately bite them on the neck or shoulder giving rise to some very nasty injuries at times.

The Nursing Staff are at their wits end to know what next to try.

They cannot in all conscience allow him to remain in his room in a solitary state, knowing as they do the seriousness of such a position. They cannot allow him always to be without clothes or bedding, even though they are aware that he will destroy them. They cannot leave him solely to his own devices. He must have human contact, he must have exercise, he must be frequently approached by Nursing Staff, and yet he responds by rejecting all such approaches and reacts as I have already described.

The Staff have attempted to dress him to take him for a walk, or to allow him the freedom of the playgrounds, all to no avail.

His mother visits daily, and he will disregard her presence and reject any attempt on her part to make contact with him.

He can and will on occasion take himself to the toilet, but there is never a day goes by without he fouls his room, or some other place.

If anyone knows of any way in which we can help this young man, then please tell us, for we are at a loss.

R. B. HUBBARD
Senior Nursing Officer

RBH/JSM

Mrs. M. Youell
S.E.N. (part-time) nights
17 February 1972

FOR THE ATTENTION OF MR. R. HUBBARD, SENIOR NURSING OFFICER. 8B.

STATEMENT—Detailed reasons for my resignation.

I have worked on Willows Villa since the second week in December, 1971, and since that time have attempted to up-grade the nursing standards. I have been repeatedly frustrated by lack of co-operation from the Charge Nurse I most frequently hand over to. The following are a few examples of what I mean:

1. I began by giving verbal and written reports to the Charge Nurse about various patients and the attention I felt they required—these reports were ignored.

2. Secondly, I drew his attention to specific patients, these include:
    i. [Patient E]—was obviously unwell and I requested him to be nursed in bed. I was given to understand, following my off-duty period, that this patient was got up and dressed. I was off Wednesday and Thursday night and this patient died Friday morning.
    ii. [Patient C]—This patient collapsed and was obviously ill, having collapsed twice during the night. I gave full nursing care and informed the N/C (who visited). Oxygen was given at intervals and patient complained of pain in the abdomen and severe spasms of coughing. He was examined next day and the diagnosis was N.A.D. No report was made on this patient by the Charge Nurse. On taking over the Villa the same night, I was concerned about him—he appeared to be in a neglected state, furred mouth, parched lips and, to me, very ill. His urinary output until 4.30 a.m. was nil and the small amount he did pass was dark and concentrated. Dr. Benton visited the ward at 5.00 a.m. to see [Patient F] and I drew her attention to [Patient C]. She examined him and recommended his transfer to the Clinic. [Patient C] died a short time later.
    iii. [Patient F]—was reported, by N/A Bartlett, to have hurt his leg at 6.30 a.m., 31 January, 1972. N/A Bartlett stated that Charge Nurse had been informed and had seen the patient. No report was made by the Charge Nurse and no Casualty form was made out. I examined patient and realised that he was seriously injured. I notified the Night Charge Nurse and was told to report verbally to Day Charge Nurse in the morning. I felt that the patient's leg was broken because of the lack of movement, swelling and abnormal rotation of the left foot. N/S informed and visited and he called Dr. Benton at about 5.00 a.m. (It was that night that Dr. Benton

186

saw [Patient C]). Following examination of [Patient F]), Dr. Benton said he was to remain in bed until X-ray and was subsequently transferred to Orsett Hospital for the treatment of a fractured femur. Report was made to Charge Nurse Large the same morning. Charge Nurse stated he didn't think there was anything wrong with him.

iv. [Patient G]—Vomited large amounts of bile, early morning Thursday 10 February. Patient looked ill and yellowish and because of his appearance and the amount of vomit, I reported this in the night report and notified my Senior Officer. I put patient back to bed. On taking over the following night, I noticed that nothing had been done regarding this patient—he died on Sunday, 13 February 1972.

v. [Patient H]—I had to really insist that this patient be brought up near the night post because he kept falling out of bed in Grand Mal Seizures. On two occasions this patient suffered serious ' G Mals ' and it was necessary to give him Paraldehyde 1/m. It is well known that his reaction to this leaves patient very unsteady on his feet and subject to falls. Charge Nurse is well aware and was told by me, but he chose to ignore the implications by getting him up after I had left.

vi. [Patient J]—Had been physically ill and advised to rest in bed on numerous occasions. Charge Nurse has agreed with me, but as soon as I have left, patient was got up and dressed and told to ' get on ' with his work. I have found patient, after taking over from Day Charge, distressed because he had been told to get up.

vii. [Patient K]—This patient has a very bad leg and N/A Bartlett has often asked me in the last few weeks to have a look at it. It was so bad on two occasions that I had to cut sock and dressing off and redress it. On one occasion, I marked dressing and it was on for four days and then I dressed it. Charge Nurse's reaction—It's a lie, his nurse does it every day.

viii. I have repeatedly asked Charge Nurse Large to re-educate the following patients and stop their brutal attacks on helpless patients in the villa:

[Patient L] ⎫ I have caught several of them punching blind
[Patient M] ⎪ and severely subnormal patients on numerous
[Patient J] ⎬ occasions and it is difficult to stop them when
[Patient N] ⎪ I am on my own with forty patients.
[Patient P] ⎭

In addition to aforementioned, Charge Nurse Large has torn up T.P.R. and B.P. charts I have made out for observations. He has also refused to take nursing notes I had made out regarding minor ailments such as rashes, boils etc, stating that all these were on the treatment book and were being dealt with, when in fact they were not—at least there was no obvious evidence of this.

Due to the above lack of co-operation and low standard of nursing care on Willows Villa, I feel that I cannot continue my work and have tendered my resignation.

(signed) M. Youell, S.E.N.

SOUTH OCKENDON GROUP HOSPITAL MANAGEMENT COMMITTEE

Members of the Hospital Management Committee as at 31 May 1972

Name and Address	Age	Appointed to Committee
Mr. W. A. Nichols, J.P. (Chairman of Hospital Management Committee)	71	April 1951
Mrs. D. A. Cloke, M.A., J.P.	67	April 1966
Mr. S. G. W. Crabb	67	February 1970
Dr. A. R. Fox, F.B.M.A., M.R.C.S., M.R.C.G.P.	72	July 1952
Dr. J. A. C. Franklin, M.B., B.S., D.P.H. County Medical Officer of Health, Essex County Council	60	April 1962
Mr. B. Glanville, F.S.V.A., F.F.S., F.R.S.H., J.P. (Vice-Chairman of Patients and Welfare Sub-Committee)	54	April 1960
Mrs. C. Godfrey	67	April 1965
Dr. G. V. Griffin, M.B., B.S., D.P.H. Medical Officer of Health, County Borough of Southend on Sea ...	43	July 1968
Mr. G. F. Howard (Chairman of Lands and Works Sub-Committee) (Vice-Chairman of Finance and General Purposes Sub-Committee) ...	52	July 1956
Mr. C. F. Mead, J.P. (Vice-Chairman of Lands and Works Sub-Committee)	67	April 1958
Mr. L. V. Norman, M.D.T.S.	(not known)	February 1971
Mr. P. J. Osborne	26	April 1972
Mrs. M. E. Protheroe (Chairman of Patients and Welfare Sub-Committee)	63	April 1962
Mr. C. R. E. Russell, LL.B.	(not known)	April 1967
Mrs. H. W. Wallis	63	September 1961

Name and Address	Age	Appointed to Committee
Mrs. F. E. Watson (Chairman of Establishment Sub-Committee)	50	April 1967
Mr. G. S. Whiting (Vice-Chairman of Hospital Management Committee) (Chairman of Finance and General Purposes Sub-Committee)	67	April 1958
Mrs. A. V. Winch, J.P. (Vice-Chairman of Establishment Sub-Committee)	(not known)	April 1966

ROYAL COLLEGE OF NURSING AND ROYAL COLLEGE OF PSYCHIATRISTS

THE CARE OF THE VIOLENT PATIENT

Extract from the Liaison Committee's Report of May 1972
The Violent Episode

19. The prevention of violence requires a knowledge and understanding of individual patients and a quiet surveillance of those factors which may precede a period of disturbed behaviour. Such signs as increasing emotional instability, changes in normal habits, anxiety, depression or bizarre behaviour ought to alert the staff to consider the cause of the change and to bring these factors to the notice of medical staff as soon as possible so that appropriate action may be taken.

20. The attitude of staff members faced with a violent episode should be calm, non-critical and non-domineering.

21. Physical confrontation should be avoided wherever possible. Talking and/or listening must be the first approach used.

22. Only as a last resort should a physical confrontation take place and only when it seems likely that someone will be hurt. Concern for property should be secondary as it can be replaced.

23. The degree of force should be the minimum required to control the violence and it should be applied in a manner that attempts to calm rather than provoke a further aggressive reaction.

24. It is only when sufficient staff are available that control of the outburst without injury to anyone involved can be achieved.

25. Clothing in preference to limbs should be used to restrain. If limbs have to be grasped they should be held near a major joint to reduce leverage and the possibility of a fracture or dislocation.
Placing the patient on the floor reduces leverage and puts the patient at a disadvantage. Shoes or boots should be removed. In exceptional circumstances, as for example when a patient is biting, the hair may have to be firmly held.

26. On no account must pressure be applied to the neck, throat, chest or abdomen.

27. If an intramuscular injection is ordered by the doctor, great care must be taken to avoid accidents in its administration.

28. Should a patient need to be segregated, it should only be for the minimum period necessary until the patient's behaviour is under control and with the consent of the doctor immediately concerned for the patient's care.

29. The patient should not be purposely avoided or treated differently afterwards, since this will only confirm his own idea of his unacceptability and perhaps further aggression.

30. It is recognised that the action suggested for dealing with violent episodes does not cover all eventualities. In some instances of extreme violence there will frequently be the need to use a considerable amount of initiative to control the patient effectively. It is in such situations where the degree of force needed becomes a matter of concern for the nurse; it is only possible to reiterate that the degree of force should be the minimum required to control the violence and it should be applied in a manner that aims to calm rather than provoke a further aggressive reaction.

Reporting Violent Episodes

31. It is essential to have an adequate reporting system. Such a system should be for the protection of any persons involved and to provide material for a critical analysis of the incident. This may suggest preventive action against future outbursts.

32. It is recognised that there is difficulty in deciding what degree of severity of violence warrants detailed reporting of the incident. The Liaison Committee consider that any of the following indications should lead to a full report:
   i. Any incident involving physical violence and injury by a patient to himself, other patients, to members of staff or to any other person.
   ii. Any incident which necessitates the use of physical restraint of a patient by members of staff.
   iii. Any incident in which segregation forms part of the management of the disturbed patient.

33. A brief account in the Ward Report is essential whether or not further reporting procedures are undertaken.

34. A report should be entered in the Nursing Notes section of the patient's case notes. This must be written by the nurse involved in the incident with any additional comments being entered by the nurse in charge of the ward.

35. The responsibility to initiate the reporting procedure should be with the nursing officer in charge of the ward, unless the patient is in the charge of some other person outside the ward at the time of the incident.

36. The principal contents of an appropriate questionnaire are listed so as to indicate the kind of information which should be recorded:
   i. When the incident occurred
   ii. Where the incident occurred
   iii. A brief factual account of the incident which should include the general activity occurring at the time of the incident
   iv. The action taken (a) Immediately
   (b) Following the incident, which should include the time that senior officers are informed and when they take action
   v. The names of all persons involved in the incident

vi. The principal content of the incident

vii. Observations on the mental state of the violent person

viii. The main direction of the aggression

ix. Any injury or damage that has occurred

x. Any additional comments on the incident.

*This list has been reproduced through the courtesy of Miss U. Budge, Principal Tutor, Tooting Bec Hospital.

37. The unit Nursing Officer should be responsible for seeing that any action needed is reported to the appropriate department of the hospital.

38. Reports on episodes of violence should finally remain in the patient's case notes.

39. Clinical notes should be kept on the ward or in a readily accessible place where the patient is resident and should contain the fullest possible information supplied by the therapeutic team so that such information may be used to facilitate treatment of the patient.

Conclusions and Recommendations

40. Even though episodes of violence in psychiatric hospitals are uncommon it is essential for all personnel who come in contact with mentally disturbed patients to acquire the necessary skills for the prevention and management of such episodes. Because of the quality of their relationship with patients psychiatric nurses will always find themselves in a vulnerable position. Adequate instruction for staff and a clear and concise reporting system are essential requisites to protect all who may be involved, patients, visitors or staff. We recommend that the Department of Health and Social Security should instruct ALL Hospital Management Committees to have a written policy for dealing with and reporting acts of violent behaviour.

192

RESIDENTIAL HOMES AND ADULT TRAINING CENTRES

Local Authority	Residential Home Places Existing	Residential Home Places Planned	Adult Training Centre Places Existing	Adult Training Centre Places Planned	Remarks
Barking: Children	—	—	120[2]		[1] 13 maintained in homes elsewhere [2] Also "sheltered workshop" for 30
Barking: Adults	50[1]	—			
Enfield: Children	20	} 40	140	170	
Enfield: Adults	20				
Hackney: Children	—	40	220		
Hackney: Adults	—	24			
Havering: Children	—	—	200		
Havering: Adults	50	60			
Haringey: Children	—	20	100	170	
Haringey: Adults	16	60			
Newham: Children	—	—	220		[3] 2 hostels planned, size not stated
Newham: Adults	—	—[3]			
Redbridge: Children	—	17	85 + [5]		[4] Plans for one other hostel [5] Also "sheltered workshop" for 40
Redbridge: Adults	12	15[4]			
Southend: Children	—	} 38	120	120	
Southend: Adults	—				
*Tower Hamlets: Children	16[6]	—	100	20	[6] Due to open August 1972
*Tower Hamlets: Adults	—	16			
Essex CC: Children	7	8	8	8	[7] None in the Thurrock area [8] No. of places in the County not stated
Essex CC: Adults	8	—			
Herts CC: Children	41	40	550	1130	
Herts CC: Adults	80	528			

* Also acts as agent for the City of London

Printed in England for Her Majesty's Stationery Office by McCorquodale Ltd.. Printers, London.
HM 7406 Dd 155929 K48 5/74.